HYPOGLYCEMIA

THE CLASSIC HEALTHCARE HANDBOOK NOW REVISED AND UPDATED

JERALDINE SAUNDERS AND DR. HARVEY M. ROSS

KENSINGTON BOOKS
http://www.kensingtonbooks.com

KENSINGTON BOOKS are published by

Kensington Publishing Corp.
850 Third Avenue
New York, NY 10022

Kensington and the K logo Reg. U.S. Pat. & TM Off.
ISBN 1-57566-064-4
First Kensington Trade Paperback Printing: August, 1996
10 9 8 7 6

Printed in the United States of America

Dedicated to
Gael
whose spirit was the real author

Special Acknowledgements

To Gaye Tardy, we express our thanks for the vision and belief in what we have to say. Her persistence and work have made it possible for others to hear us.

—J.S. and H.M.R.

To Arthur R. Andrews, my husband, for all his help and support with this project.

—J.S.

To Jan-Michael Kennedy, my thanks for his unselfish contributions, which have made this a better book than it would have been without him.

—H.M.R.

Grateful acknowledgement is also given J. L. Courtney of the Lee Foundation, W. D. Currier, M.D., Stig R. Erlander, Ph.D., Rob Krakovitz, M.D., Fred Rohe, and R. Stanton for permission to use their material in this work.

The inferior doctor treats actual illness;
The mediocre doctor cures imminent illness;
The superior doctor prevents illness.

—Old Chinese Proverb

A healthy body is a bounteous host to the soul,
A sick body, its prison.

—Francis Bacon

Contents

Notes from the Authors

Traditional medicine is facing an upheaval as vast numbers of people across the nation are becoming increasingly aware of its inadequacies. Fed up with patch-and-mend medicine that treats symptoms but does little to prevent or cure disease, people are looking for innovative and safe alternatives. Let us get to the business of preventive medicine and healing now.

Jeraldine Saunders

Medicine as it is generally practiced today is often helpful, sometimes harmful, and almost always limited in scope. If I needed an operation, I'd want to see a surgeon, not a nutritionist. If I had a broken bone, I'd want an orthopedist to be the first one to administer to me. And if I had a heart attack, I'd want to be in the hands of an expert cardiologist. Many of these physicians practice their art well. I only hope that in administering to me I am one of the lucky ones who do not end up with an illness caused by the treatment, an all-too-frequent situation.

The limits of medicine should not be criticized, for who or what is not limited? However, failure to recognize such limitations should not only be criticized but is reprehensible.

The importance of nutrition is almost universally ignored

by the practicing physician today. Sometimes it is not ignored but scorned or dismissed with "eat properly and you get everything you need." With some exceptions, this is true, but what is "eating properly"? The average physician cannot tell you. Even this is acceptable. But what is not acceptable is that he is unaware that he doesn't know. He doesn't want to know what it is he doesn't know. With such a beginning, there is nowhere to go.

While physicians are indispensable and as a group contribute greatly to the health of the sick, so much more could be done to help the ill become healthier, and to enable the healthy to maintain that state. At any one time, the majority of the population is well, yet most of the effort and resources of the medical profession are directed toward the ill. Only cursory attention is given to the well to enable them to maintain their good health.

This book is not intended to insult the vast majority of talented physicians who practice their art daily and in so doing restore health and relieve suffering. Yet it is hoped that some physicians, either in reading a book such as this or in being inspired by their patients, will eventually say to themselves, "Perhaps there is another way."

Harvey M. Ross, M.D.

Preface

It is an alarming fact that countless Americans suffer—unsuspectingly—from the debilitating effects of hypoglycemia, a diet-related condition caused by low blood sugar. Unless the symptoms are diagnosed, a multitude of mental and physical disorders can go undetected.

According to Rob Krakovitz, M.D., who specializes in metabolic nutrition, "In the United States today, in my estimation, approximately fifty percent of the population experience symptoms related to blood sugar fluctuations. These include fatigue, depression, irritability, headaches, poor memory, and many others."

Moreover, research has shown that low blood sugar may cause such common conditions as epilepsy, multiple sclerosis, peptic ulcers, asthma, alcoholism, allergies, heart attacks, drug addiction, and cancer. The childhood disease rheumatic fever may also have its origins in a hypoglycemic condition, and there is no doubt that there is a relationship between mental illness and low blood sugar; tests conducted by hundreds of doctors have borne this out.

However, much of the medical establishment still refuses to recognize nutrition as an important therapeutic tool in the treatment of disease. By their very refusal, doctors themselves have made hypoglycemia the disease your doctor won't treat.

Most doctors are unable to detect hypoglycemia because few have learned that they, when testing for the disease, must consider individual differences. What is a low level of blood sugar for one person may not be low for another. The rate at which the blood sugar is falling must also be considered.

It is too easy for a physician, even one who is conscious of the value of nutrition as a therapeutic tool, to fall into the accepted mode for treating disease. It is too easy for any United States-trained physician, accustomed to concentrating on crisis intervention, to forget that a more important far-reaching goal of medicine is to keep the healthy, healthy.

Among Dr. Ross's own patients, about 95 percent of them want treatments for problems. Only a small percentage come to him and say, "I'm healthy. I want to stay that way. Is there any advice you can give me?"

The best treatment, however, is prevention. Hypoglycemia can usually be prevented if a person pays attention to his or her diet. And in so doing, there's a good chance that many other diseases will be prevented as well.

This book provides a much-needed perspective on a large number of diseases that have a common cause—the grossly improper American diet—and the nutritional treatments that have proven to be of great help in their management.

It is intended for *everyone:* those who want to maintain good health; those who have hypoglycemia; those who want to prevent it and other conditions; and all those who want to know how to eat well, get well, and *stay* well.

PART I
GAEL

Chapter One

Please, Doctor, Help!

The baby was furiously active in the womb, much more active than the thin, tall, malnourished 96-pound teenager who would give birth to it. Drained of strength, the young mother often wondered if she could endure the final weeks of waiting. It had been a difficult pregnancy compounded by her undetected malnutrition and the fact that her husband was overseas fighting in World War II. She did so wish that he could be with her at this time.

The culmination of the birth cycle was not easy, either, for the placenta had separated; the delivery was by Caesarian section. The operation was performed successfully, however, and even though the doctor had been sure the baby would be a boy, since there were such active prenatal movements, it was a beautiful girl with blue eyes and blonde hair. And at 3:20 P.M., on that December 6, 1943, she was named Gael.

Because the mother was so malnourished and the birth premature, there was no breast milk, so the mother followed the doctor's recommendations for baby formula. She bought the prepared powder for the formula at the drugstore and obediently mixed it with Karo syrup. She thought this was a poor substitute for mother's milk, but she had no reason to question it; this was before women found out the importance of breast-feeding. She would have preferred to breast-feed, but her doctor had assured her that Gael would do well on the formula. Yet the baby didn't thrive. Although Gael looked fine and gained normal amounts of weight, there was something terribly wrong. Little Gael couldn't sleep well; she was the victim of a terrifying insomnia.

When the mother confronted the doctor with this problem, he laughed. "That's impossible," he said, "babies don't have insomnia!" In 1943, medical doctors knew even less about nutrition than they do today. The bewildered young mother listened to the doctor's words, but they didn't change the fact that Gael couldn't sleep well. The mother found herself massaging her baby's tiny back for long hours at a time so that Gael could at least have a few hours of fitful sleep. But Gael's condition did not get better. When she was two and three, she was the only child in the neighborhood who couldn't fall asleep for an afternoon nap. She would toss and turn before dropping off at night. She was always operating at full speed and, we realize now, was actually hyperkinetic. This term for hyperactive children was unheard of then.

By this time, the mother's health once more was a problem, and her husband, who had never adapted well to child-rearing, was beginning to drink heavily. But even though the mother was suffering with stomach ulcers, she never shirked her duties. She read every book about babies that she could get her hands on, and every magazine article about their care that she could find time for. But in those days, the books and magazines were far from enlightening on the subject of good nutrition. She also looked for help by reading books on child psychology. She spent long hours in the kitchen baking cookies, cakes, and pies—the things she and her husband and Gael liked to eat. (Just like the perfect mother that Madison Avenue projected in books and magazines.) She was trying hard, but since she was unenlightened, she felt she was doing the right things in following that era's misinformation.

Gael seemed healthy as a youngster except for being hyperactive, and she adapted readily to school. Her mother had been concerned earlier—especially over such alarming developments as baby teeth coming in with decay spots—but here was Gael, in school and at the top of her class. She was beautiful, talented, and exceptionally bright, with a photographic memory.

During the long night hours when sleep eluded her, she would memorize the stories her mother read to her and proudly recite them in class the next day. And whenever there was a school play, Gael was awarded the leading role.

She didn't get much sleep, but she seemed able to get along without it. Nonetheless, her mother worried about the insomnia and Gael's frequent bouts with bronchitis and the need to be rescued with antibiotics. She missed school a great deal because of this, but the sympathetic teachers in grammar school were always more than willing to allow her to make up her tests at her leisure.

Gael loved her early years in school. An only child, she thrived on her friendships in the classroom. She was a sweet and sensitive child, someone quite special, and she easily maintained a straight-A average in her studies.

Then something went wrong. The change took place when Gael passed through puberty, at about 11.

By this time, her mother was doing well as a model, a job she chose because it allowed her to work part-time and to be there when Gael got home from school. The family moved into a lovely house with a pool, but Gael didn't enjoy the home as much as her mother expected. Gael began to withdraw into herself. When friends would come to swim, she would go off to her room to be alone. She dropped all outside activities, such as Girl Scouts, and spent all her time studying. She maintained her grades, but she changed from an extrovert to an introvert. She showed no interest in dancing or dating and became a total enigma to family and friends. This was a particularly bad time for Gael's mother. By now, her ulcers were so bad that she was being hospitalized three or four times a year. And Gael's father had left because of his heavy drinking. The mother consulted many doctors, but none of them helped her, her husband, or Gael. She was desperate for some answer.

Finally, when Gael was about 14, her mother found a book entitled *Body, Mind, and Sugar,* by Dr. E.M. Abrahamson and

A.W. Pezet, which contained statistics proving that low blood sugar could be the cause of over- or underweight, fatigue, allergies, bronchitis, schizophrenia, asthma, alcoholism, depression, peptic and duodenal ulcers, migraine headaches, suicide, and even murder. After she read the book, it became alarmingly clear to her that low blood sugar could account not only for her own ulcers, as well as her husband's alcoholism, but also for Gael's prenatal activity, since such activity occurs if the mother is malnourished. It explained Gael's hyperactivity, her insomnia, her bronchial attacks, and her reclusiveness. The mother was certain she now had the answer, but the question was what should she do with it? She took the book to her own loving family who lived nearby. It failed to impress them. From the family doctor? The same reaction. It is human nature to react to new ideas first by laughing, then later, maybe years later, by considering, and maybe much later on, by accepting. She attempted to impress Gael with information and was dubbed a "health nut," a term Gael had learned at school to describe anyone interested in nutrition. The mother was neatly labeled an eccentric, and Gael went on eating destructively from the school vending machines and lunch counters.

Like most teenagers who have hypoglycemia, 14-year-old Gael was not easy to handle. She refused to accept her mother's "idiosyncracies" about health, especially since her own doctor also disagreed with her mother. She ate what nourishing foods her mother could disguise adequately, but refused to eat the necessary frequent, small nutritious meals; nor would she follow a diet low in refined carbohydrates. Gael was encouraged to resist since she was told by teachers, friends, and her doctors that "low blood sugar" was just a fad. When her mother prepared tasty desserts, Gael would ask, "Is this real food or pretend food?" If it was made without sugar (hypoglycemics cannot have sugar), she would refuse to eat it. Suspicious of her mother's tricks, and afraid of being manipulated, she ate hardly anything at home. The junk foods at school gave her the taste she was accustomed to.

It was in 1957 that Gael's mother started eliminating all

refined carbohydrates from her diet, as explained in *Body, Mind, and Sugar,* and it marked the end of her own health difficulties. Her ulcers disappeared, never to return. She gained the proper weight to fill out her 5-foot, 7-inch frame, and her energy increased proportionately. The results she obtained sufficiently motivated her to commence studying nutrition seriously. She has continued to study until the present day.

With knowledge gained from her studying, she launched a diet campaign that would restore her health for the rest of her life, but much as she tried, she could not sell the diet to her doctor, to Gael, to the rest of her family, or to her daughter's long line of doctors. Gael's greatest troubles were about to begin.

Gael graduated from junior high school with honor grades and entered high school as reclusive as she had been during puberty. She had a very sensitive, lovable personality and was very popular, yet she accepted hardly any dates and retired to her room each evening "to study." Determined to be chosen orator of her tenth-grade class, she wrote an extraordinarily fine speech that she memorized perfectly and was awarded the honor of representing her class. When it came her turn to speak, she delivered the address perfectly, too. It may have been the last real accomplishment Gael realized in school. The strain of her condition seemed to drain her of determination, rob her of incentive, deplete her strength, and increase the severity of her mood swings.

It was all her mother could do to keep Gael operating sufficiently to finish the next two years of high school. She missed many days because of bronchial difficulties, common in some hypoglycemics, and missed almost as many days because of exhaustion or lack of energy, another symptom of hypoglycemia.

At the end of Gael's second year of high school, her mother had to have her transferred to a professional school where absences would not affect her grades. The public school could not pass students who were absent too much, no matter how good their grades were. Gael's IQ had not dropped; only her energy had. If it was a matter of making up tests, she did so readily and got straight As.

When she was 15, because she had such excellent grades, Gael was admitted as a special student to summer school at the University of California at Santa Barbara, about a three-hour drive from her home. She enjoyed the summer of special studies and the freedom it gave her. Living in the dormitory was fun, and she made lots of new friends, but after eating lots of junk foods and making frequent use of the Coke machines in the dorm, she returned early when a bronchial attack incapacitated her.

Once again, Gael's doctors all agreed with her that her mother was a "health nut," that vitamins and hypoglycemia were just fads, that her bronchitis had nothing to do with low blood sugar, and that vitamins were not important. These doctors were simply ignorant about nutrition, hypoglycemia, and preventive medicine.

When it came time for her to go to college, Gael had ideas of her own. She wanted to study law at George Washington University in Washington, D.C., far from her California home. She remained there a year and a half, until she was flown home after a bout with bronchial pneumonia and the usual doses of antibiotics. Subsequently, she attended USC, and later UCLA, but she simply did not have as much energy as her fellow students. She had a passion for education and loved to study, and she did so want to please her mother by being able to graduate, but she couldn't keep up the pace physically or emotionally.

Whenever Gael was taken to the doctor because of her energy swings, her mother begged for confirmation about her theories. The physicians only shrugged and gave Gael understanding winks. They had been warned about her food-freaky mother. "Your daughter is fine," they would insist. "There is nothing wrong with her." For Gael's chronic insomnia, they would give her prescriptions for tranquilizers and sleeping pills, and send her on her way. Time and time again, different doctors said she was fine. Even those doctors who were forced to test her blood sugar said that she was okay since they did not know how to read the results of the glucose tolerance test. (This test and how to interpret it will be discussed later on in this book.) It was actually quite obvious from Gael's glucose tolerance tests that there was a rapid decline in her blood sugar during the second hour of each test. But the interpretations were made only by doctors who couldn't, or wouldn't, recognize hypoglycemia.

It is true that outwardly Gael did not look ill, which perhaps was to her disadvantage. In fact, she looked bright, healthy, and incredibly beautiful. Warner Brothers Studios was interested in signing her for films, she was frequently asked to be in beauty contests, and she was approached with work as a junior model. Gael accepted several such opportunities. However, she always had to give up. She would be filled with enthusiasm at the outset of a new movie, but after a day or a day and a half of work, she would come home, overcome by stress and tension. Never really sick enough to be in bed, but still not energetic enough to work, she began to feel guilty over her failure to hold a job. She meant well and sincerely wanted to remove the burden of her mother's support. She was 24 years old at this time.

Then the answer for her seemed to present itself. She met a young man. She became infatuated, and when he asked her to marry him, she accepted.

But this, too, was a terrible failure. Her inexperienced husband couldn't begin to cope with a beautiful young woman who failed in what he felt were her wifely duties and, moreover, never slept. The marriage was brief. Gael was now 25. She still hadn't gotten any help from the long line of physicians. All they did was prescribe coverup drugs: tranquilizers, sleeping pills. She never had the slightest difficulty in getting prescriptions from any of the doctors she visited, but not once asked what her eating habits were or mentioned the importance of nutrition or knew how to recognize subclinical malnutrition or hypoglycemia.

Because the brain is critically dependent on circulating glucose, great fluctuations can lead to serious shifts in mood. As a result of this biochemical imbalance, Gael's relationship with her mother worsened. Gael felt guilty about what she felt were her failures, and this manifested itself in hostility toward her mother.

To ease the tension between them, her mother accepted a position on a luxury liner as a cruise director. She felt it might be better to leave Gael on her own for a time, to give her more freedom and allow her to have her mother's apartment to herself. She wouldn't be far from family, either. Gael's grandmother and uncle lived next door, if they were needed.

Between each 12- to 14-day cruise, the mother would return to find Gael ignoring her diet and even more disdainful of her mother's advice. Her mother tried to reason with her, using her own health as an example. The mother was now in her mid-forties and she would point out that even though she often worked 15 hours a day, and in spite of her own hypoglycemia and the demands of the job, she always felt strong and energetic. By eliminating refined carbohydrates and by maintaining a good nutritional diet, she was able to cope, she said. Everyone, including doctors, assured Gael that her mother was still a food faddist, a health freak, a nutritional nut. And Gael's biochemical balance was so off that she couldn't have been reasoned with anyway. The mother's anguish at being unable to get help for her daughter gave her a heavy heart indeed, which became greater each time she was unable to find help.

It seemed as if a psychic premonition propelled the mother to rush home from one of her cruises. She felt something was wrong; she knew it. She fumbled with the keys in the front door and worried when there was no response to her knocking. Gael was inside. She was sure of it, but why was there no answer? Once inside, she ran frantically to the bathroom as though a hand was guiding her. There was Gael, on the floor, unconscious. She had fallen against the tub. All her upper teeth were broken off, and the upper jaw was apparently fractured. Had she fallen because tranquilizers had caused her to have a low blood sugar blackout?

After she had brought Gael to, the mother took her to

three oral surgeons who had seemed willing to answer the emergency call when she'd called them on the telephone. But they all backed out when Gael came staggering into their offices. Frantically, the mother drove Gael to a pair of hospitals, but she was refused emergency assistance because of her vertigo-like condition. In addition, Gael was beginning to become belligerent. Unable to recognize a victim of hypoglycemia, the doctors advised that the only facility that would accommodate such a case was Olive View, located far in the San Fernando Valley. This was a small psychiatric hospital and the only hope left. Desperate by this time, the mother started driving, with Gael slumped next to her in the car seat. She dreaded having her daughter wake up for fear of the questions. If they were answered, there would be anger. She hoped Gael would sleep. The mother had only 24 hours before she had to sail again. If she lost her job, she and Gael would be helpless.

As they drove through the silent streets, the mother worried that she might miss the proper turn off. She prayed for help. She wanted nothing to arouse Gael's suspicions. If Gael got the idea she was headed for a psychiatric hospital, she would certainly become hysterical. The same guiding hand that drew the mother home and into the bathroom directed her to the hospital. The staff could not have been more cooperative.

To expedite Gael's admission, she was left in the car while her mother went inside to register her. When the task was complete, the mother returned to the car for her daughter. She was gone. The car was empty.

After an hour's search, Gael was found, hidden in a clump of bushes. She required restraint, but finally was admitted.

Gael's inborn fear of psychiatric hospitals even then was understandable. Recent studies have shown that medication is often the sole form of treatment and is sometimes used merely to control unruly patients. The drugs themselves are suspected of causing the very psychosis they are supposed to treat. Psychiatric patients are given drugs without their informed consent, often by intramuscular injection if they refuse to take it orally. Where are their human rights?

Visitors to large mental hospitals have become so used to the patients' strange gait that it is now commonly called the "thorazine shuffle." Treating mental illness, especially schizophrenia, with drugs instead of correcting the diet and testing for candidiasis, is not only useless but criminal. "Zonking" patients out with drugs is not only unproductive and harmful but causes additional iatrogenic illness, caused by the treatment itself.

In Gael's case, the mother pleaded with the personnel at the hospital to please not give her daughter *any* medication.

They must have listened to her because Gael was patched together physically, and over the next three months made progress in combatting her dependence on the tranquilizers and sleeping pills her doctors had been prescribing. Gael liked the hospital and admitted that it was helping her, even though she still had no energy. Paradoxically, however, when she was examined by the authorities after the required time period, she said she wanted to go home. She spoke cogently and convinced them that she was ready to leave. They agreed. Her hypoglycemia—the cause of her problems—hadn't been cured though.

Each time her mother returned from a cruise, Gael's mood swings were more extreme and she was unable to work, yet everyone assured the mother that Gael was fine. Wasn't she up and about and looking beautiful, as usual? She was eating everything that was wrong for her and so was unable to sleep and again was taking her doctor's advice and taking sleeping pills and tranquilizers. This continued until one day, several months later, when a telephone call stopped the mother as she was about to embark on a cruise to the Mediterranean. The call was from Gael's uncle, who informed her that Gael had been found in her bed. She had "passed on." Was it from an overdose of sleeping pills taken accidentally in her search for relief from the terrifying insomnia that had plagued her since infancy? Or was it from hypoglycemic shock? No difference, really. Either way, the cause was the same.

It was unbearable for the mother. In her mind, she kept hearing herself talking to all those doctors throughout the years. One after another, they had refused to gather the facts to analyze correctly the problem before them. Gael had wandered through countless consultation rooms, but was unable to survive the faulty diagnoses. They had prescribed more and different drugs, and had failed. In response to the anguished mother, they asked, *"Where is your license to practice medicine? Oh, you haven't got one? Then how dare you think you know more than we doctors do."* They believed they had learned everything in medical school, but they had caused the death of another innocent victim.

After Gael's funeral, the mother went home. The refrigerator was filled with colas, sweet rolls, cakes—everything a hypoglycemic should not have but craves. She looked in the medicine chest. There were the sleeping pills—enough to put her daughter to sleep forever, even if a first accidental overdose failed. She cried out, "Why?" How could it have happened? Weren't there laws about filling potentially fatal barbiturate prescriptions? No. There were no such laws at that time. The pharmacist was required to fill the prescription written by a physician, and the physician could write as many prescriptions as he wanted to. *It's big business!* They were sorry, she was sure, but it was done.

She kept remembering how, in spite of her pleas, the pills kept rolling in. In fact, her desperate attempt to have the police help was to no avail. From desk sergeant to detective, the words were the same, "Lady, if I were you, I'd leave the matter alone. The doctors know what they are doing."

There are hundreds of such stories, I'm sure, but, unfortunately, I know this one best and I know it is true. It's one I personally lived through, for Gael was my daughter.

Chapter Two

The Magnificent Minority

Digging deeper for the truth, one would be forced to conclude that Gael was yet another sacrifice to apathy in the field of preventive medicine. Gael died at the age of 27, a victim of hypoglycemia, some would say. I would say that she was a victim of the Dark Ages of biochemistry.

I learned to live with my grief and to reconstruct my life—a life that would allow me to continue to search for truth in the areas of nutrition, biochemistry, and hypoglycemia, and also to communicate and share that truth through lecturing, as I had been doing for several years on cruise ships.

My favorite lecture was called "Vim and Vigor." It was a health talk that lured passengers into the ship's theater in their search for what appeared to be my secret for a trim figure and a zest for life. After we had sailed out to sea, the laws of the land didn't apply any longer, so I was then free to relate the latest findings in the field of preventive medicine. The passengers loved the talk and would take home my printed diet. The huge amounts of mail I received when my ship returned to home port was amazing. Not only was I stunned by the number of letters, but by the accounts of the glowing experiences of new-found health that the passengers gained when they followed the diet (found later on in this book). I wish I had the space to share some of the beautiful stories I received from these correspondents.

The tragedy Gael and I suffered would not be in vain, I felt, if I could be instrumental in preventing similar future horrors.

I continue to lecture, not only on ships, but on land, too, to keep the latest biochemical and general health findings flowing to as many ears as I can reach.

I was even able to slip ideas on nutrition and its importance into my first book, my autobiography, *The Love Boats* (Pinnacle Books, Inc., N.Y., 1975), which is about what really happens above and below decks on cruise ships; it became a successful best-seller and TV series.

I continue to speak, to listen, to write, to make inquiries, to learn by teaching, to synthesize what I have learned with what I am learning. The experience I had with Gael prods me on. Imagine my anguish when I see young, loving mothers buying Cokes, Twinkies, and candies for their children. When will we require proper nutrition classes for all high school students, not only to help them but to help their offspring?

I bring to this writing almost 20 years of serious, dedicated research and experience in the field of nutrition, preventive medicine, and biochemistry. I write from a background of intensive participation. I have trained myself to discern the differences between fact, theory, and blind adherence to orthodox beliefs.

Professionals and laymen who once had "hermetically" sealed minds and attitudes are now being given platforms to decry the harmful effects of processed foods on our bodies. My views are being vindicated, and although it is too late to help Gael, it is not too late to help the other "Gaels" of this world.

It was during my mission that I encountered for the second time a physician named Harvey M. Ross. When I heard his words coming from the stage of the huge auditorium at the conference of the International College of Applied Nutrition, I realized why it was filled with his followers, plus a long waiting line at the entrance. He certainly was the guru for the "new thought" in the medical field. At this writing, he is vice-president of the Academy of Orthomolecular Psychiatry, and secretary-treasurer of the International College of Applied Nutrition. He is now recognized as one of the world's most informed doctors on hypoglycemia and biochemistry.

At this particular lecture, he was discussing his therapeutic methods and his newest findings. As I continued to listen, I thanked God that there was a full house to hear this brave man.

Ironically, I thought to myself, wouldn't it have been wonderful to have encountered this tall, handsome genius during Gael's long road of suffering? As he continued to talk, it was as though I was seeing through trick mirrors, as if I was seeing two Doctor Rosses. In one mirror, I was seeing this dedicated, informed individual carrying a spear in a crusade for truth. In the other mirror, I was seeing the same lanky body, the same intelligent face, but the words were strangely different. And the time was not now, but many years ago when this same Dr. Ross—whom Gael had a "crush" on—declared to Gael and me, eager for help, "Mrs. Saunders, there is nothing wrong with Gael that has anything to do with nutrition, vitamins, low blood sugar, etc., etc." All the accepted, traditional rhetoric was being repeated to me again. "That's right, Mother," Gael was saying. "Now will you stop paying so much attention to what I eat? Please?"

As much as I shook my head, deliberately blanked my mind, and attempted to reassemble the picture, it was the same Dr. Ross only in a different time slot. Yes! He was one of the doctors who could have prevented my daughter's tragedy and did not because he, like so many others, unfortunately, was *then* a victim of his own orthodox training with all its accompanying preconceived academic prejudices and lack of knowledge about treating the mind and body as one. Yes, I was sure now that this great man was one of those doctors in the passing parade of failures whom Gael and I had encountered in our search for help. And this was also the same doctor whom I drove miles to listen to because of the giant strides he had made in helping hypoglycemics and in becoming one of the first orthomolecular psychiatrists.

Dr. Ross came upon the biochemical approach by accident. He was working as staff physician at Gracie Square Psychiatric Hospital in Manhattan, after residencies at the New York State Psychiatric Institute and the New York Veterans Administration hospitals. All his background and experience had been extremely analytically oriented. Gracie Square attracted patients who were either severely depressed or schizophrenic in emergency situations. He became acquainted with Dr. Allan Cott by telephone, since Cott often referred patients to Gracie Square for emergency treatment. Ross admits he thought Cott something of a fanatic with his emphasis on diet and vitamins, but Ross was soon converted himself.

Before Dr. Cott went on vacation for several weeks, he asked Dr. Ross to take over his practice until his return. When patients forgot or neglected to follow Dr. Cott's prescribed dosage of vitamins and diet, the reaction was dramatic. Ross decided he would either have to ignore all the evidence or join him. He elected to join with Cott. He resigned from Gracie Square and teamed up with Dr. Cott for three years. Now, Dr. Ross is one of the magnificent minority in the field of nutrition and biochemistry, which is why I chose him to be my co-author. He, like everyone else who takes on an "avant garde" approach to new ideas in medicine, must tolerate his colleagues' fears of the unconventional. It can be a stain on one's character that is not easily removed.

We understand and hold no bitterness toward people who cling with parochial steadfastness to the belief that the sick of body or mind are strictly the province of the drug-oriented pill pushers in the medical field.

The public must be protected, it is agreed, but not at the cost of our freedom to discover something of great value. I'm certain that almost everyone will agree that being a member of the illustrious American Medical Association does not automatically confer total knowledge in the art of healing.

Remember the ridicule the late Linus Pauling received when he first tried to convince the medical field of the importance and value of vitamin C? The *laughing and considering* stages are over and finally we are enjoying the benefits of the *acceptance* stage. What a pity it would have been if Linus Pauling had been denied the right to delve into a technical and complicated area of research because he was not an M.D.

PART II

THE DISEASE YOUR DOCTOR WON'T TREAT

Chapter Three

Hypoglycemia—The Fad Disease?

Ruth's marriage had almost been ruined. She was furious. Anne's marriage had been ruined. She was bewildered.

Derek was too irritable to be promoted and had never reached his professional potential. He was angry.

Frank was too tired to work. He was resigned to not trying anything but a monotonous job that required no thinking and a minimum of energy.

The question they all had a few months later, after they had been diagnosed as hypoglycemics and were showing improvement was "Why didn't my doctor do anything years ago when I first started complaining?"

One can only surmise that large numbers of people needlessly suffer year after year because of hypoglycemia. Numerous people have been through my office, with histories of years of treatment for depression, anxiety, fatigue, with little or no results because the cause wasn't being treated. There are numerous instances in which patients were not given anything for their complaints because their laboratory reports indicated they were well. If the laboratory test results are normal, it is assumed that no legitimate illness exists. How much suffering could have been avoided; how much time could have been saved if a proper glucose tolerance test had been done, followed by a proper interpretation of the test and correct treatment.

The diagnosis and treatment of hypoglycemia is a medical disgrace. The diagnosis is not complicated, yet day after day, year after year, people suffer because their doctors did not diagnose and treat the condition properly.

I don't know why it is true, but hypoglycemia is a disease your doctor won't treat. To be perfectly accurate, we should say "probably won't treat," because there are physicians who recognize this illness and treat it properly. These physicians are often scorned by the medical establishment. Too many times I have seen people with sad, tired faces who had the same story of not feeling well, of feeling tired and having no stamina, and yet they had been pronounced healthy by a myriad of physicians. Too many times the patient had suggested to the doctor that the root of the problem might be hypoglycemia. And too many times the suffering patient was rebuffed with "there is no such thing as hypoglycemia," or "I don't believe in hypoglycemia." At least these physicians were out in the open and straightforward in their rebuffs and did not care whether prejudices were showing. Unfortunately, some doctors underestimate the intelligence of their patients and try to pacify them by doing inadequate testing. This is dishonest. Other times, a lack of information or a misinterpretation of data lead to the conclusion, "You're okay. You don't have hypoglycemia."

A Los Angeles television news program produced a short segment on hypoglycemia. The problem of obtaining a proper diagnosis was raised. When asked, one of the panelists commented, "Provided you can get your physician to do the proper testing, the chance of a proper diagnosis is about 5 percent." In my experience this is an accurate estimate.

Much is good about American medicine in spite of the lackluster figures we read on the health of the American people as compared to people in some other countries. The attitude of physicians concerning hypoglycemia is a small part of the total picture of medical care, but it is an important area where extremists contribute little and only look foolish. Not every disease is hypoglycemia, and neither will every disease be cured by an extreme dose of vitamins. On the other hand, to dismiss this disease with "I don't believe in hypoglycemia" is incomprehensibly arrogant in anyone, and especially in scientists. If someone said, "I don't believe in poverty," "I don't believe in man's inhumanity to man," "I don't believe in wars," or "I don't believe in suffering," no matter who the authority was and no matter how strongly it was stated, the condition would not vanish. Similarly, the disbelief of one physician or the entire medical society will not make hypoglycemia disappear, either.

Patients have a variety of experiences with their doctors, of course, ranging from the proper treatment to the attitude that hypoglycemia is only a fad. As a matter of fact, it seems that it's now a fad to label hypoglycemia a fad disease. This label, which is sometimes applied by otherwise competent, respected authorities, is all that is necessary to convince a small but important group of physicians that they need not consider a "nonexistent" disease. They need only cite the authority to diminish the curiosity of the patient who suspects hypoglycemia. Such statements, made by those who should know better, probably have caused years of unnecessary suffering for those patients who were unable to obtain proper treatment. It is curious that those same physicians argue that overdiagnosing a fad disease has made patients out of those who should not be patients and has prevented those who blame their problems on hypoglycemia from getting the "proper treatment," presumably psychotherapy.

One begins to doubt whether these authorities have ever been patients who after years of psychotherapy find that their major problem is what they have been eating, not what they have been thinking, not their poor interpersonal relationships, and not their poor self-esteem, all of which are the result of years of living with untreated hypoglycemia. Treating the psychological symptoms of hypoglycemia without treating hypoglycemia itself is like treating a headache caused by a brain tumor with an aspirin.

Some of the patients who have seen doctors who told them that hypoglycemia did not exist related truly astounding tales. When reviewing a glucose tolerance curve that had figures well below that which is ordinarily classed as indicating hypoglycemia, a doctor stated, "Well, you see, since there is no such thing as hypoglycemia, we'll have to look further into what caused this." A statement that obviously makes no sense is usually not worth stating.

Another doctor told his patient, "There is no such thing as hypoglycemia, but if you insist, we can do a five-hour glucose tolerance test to prove it." Would you subject yourself to such a test if the person who is going to interpret the results has given you his interpretation before he has done the test?

Other physicians who are less adamant and who are willing to recognize hypoglycemia fail in the diagnosis because of the strict guidelines they use in interpreting the results of the glucose test. These guidelines assume that there is one blood sugar level above which a person is well and below which a person has hypoglycemia. Any schoolchild with an average intelligence can recognize basic individual differences. Some people sleep six hours, some sleep eight hours; some eat 3,000 calories a day, some 2,000. How could there possibly be one blood sugar level for everyone below which a person would exhibit hypoglycemic symptoms and above which the person would function well?

Another major problem preventing the correct interpretation of the test results is that most physicians do not observe their patients or ask them about their reactions during the glucose tolerance test. At times, these observations are essential in making the correct diagnosis. I have seen patients whose symptoms have been so severe at a point during the glucose tolerance test that the test was stopped, and yet the physician did not make a diagnosis of hypoglycemia because the results obtained by the laboratory did not fit into the narrow criteria being used. To make a diagnosis after examining only the laboratory figures, as is done most of the time, breaks one of the fundamental rules of medicine: "Treat the patient." In this time of advancing technology, too often medicine treats the laboratory reports and not the patient.

Patients often ask me why their doctors have such a negative attitude toward hypoglycemia. I don't know, but I can guess. Man's recorded history of science is full of similar examples of slow acceptance of new ideas. Two well-known examples are Lister's Germ Theory of Disease and Semmelweiss's insistence on the physician's need to scrub his hands before delivering a child or examining an expectant mother. In both instances, there was a clear need for more knowledge to unravel some of the mysteries of the fatal illnesses of the time. Yet even with the clear need, the established physicians and professional organizations not only did not accept the new theories, but ridiculed and tried to discourage the theories' originators. Another well-known example, Dr. Sigmund Freud, experienced similar treatment for years at the hands of his colleagues.

It is interesting to note that American medicine was not always critical when it came to hypoglycemia. Dr. Seale Harris, who first described the condition, was treated with respect and given recognition by his colleagues in the mid 1920s for his work in bringing to light this condition. In the early 1920s, doctors were gaining experience with a newly available hormone, insulin, in their treatment of diabetes. Dr. Seale Harris reasoned that if diabetes was a disease in which not enough insulin was produced, thus causing a high sugar level in the blood, then there might be a disease in which too much insulin is produced, causing a low blood sugar level. A characteristic reaction was noted when too much insulin was given. An overdose of insulin would lower the blood sugar and cause hunger, tremors, sweating, and perhaps fainting. He observed that some patients had similar symptoms to those people who had been given too much insulin. For no apparent reason, these patients would have tremors, perspire profusely, and feel weak and confused. Following up his suspicions with laboratory tests, Dr. Harris uncovered patients who had very low blood sugar levels. He eventually learned that these patients responded to a low carbohydrate diet and that many of them had to eat frequently. Even today, the Seale Harris diet remains the basis for the traditional treatment of hypoglycemia.

Physicians in the 1920s recognized hypoglycemia as a disease with multiple symptoms, both medical and psychological. However, after the medical profession's initial interest, Dr. Harris's work was quickly forgotten.

Perhaps part of the current problem is that hypoglycemia was reintroduced in nonmedical literature. This led many patients to go to their physicians asking to be tested for the condition. Most doctors are put off by self-diagnosis, by a breakdown in the traditional doctor-patient relationship. I know, I'm a doctor. Many physicians do not like patients telling them what to look for, especially if the examinations have not uncovered sufficient reasons for the patient's complaints. In the minds of many physicians, such a breakdown in the traditional role-playing is detrimental to the patient-physician relationship. The physician clings to the role of the potent, "all knowing" professional, and in so doing, hopes to retain the respect of his patient.

Forty or 50 years ago, when there was little else to use in medicine to effect a cure, such strength, determination, and bull-headedness was transmitted positively to the patient, relatives and friends and was therapeutic. Many scientific, technical, moral, and social changes have taken place in the past 50 years, many within the last 20. The attitude of most patients toward their physician has also changed. Most patients today value honesty in their relationship with their physician. They do not want predigested, performed dogma handed to them. They want a physician who is informed in the proven methods, but one who is also willing to be open-minded in some newer areas where help might be obtained. Patients want to be able to believe their physician when he says, "I know," and the belief can only be there if the physician is capable of saying "I don't know" when he doesn't. No one expects another person to be informed equally in all areas, but it is fair to expect the expert to know the areas of his own strengths and weaknesses and to have the honesty to direct his patients within those limitations.

Another problem in the treatment of hypoglycemia is that, for the most part, hypoglycemia is not very exciting to physicians who become much more intrigued with obscure diseases with equally obscure names. Hypoglycemics have no obvious tumors or medical illnesses, and the treatment is nutritional. The extent of the average physician's lack of information about nutrition is scandalous. I have heard Dr. Carlton Fredricks, noted nutritionist and lecturer, state quite appropriately, "The average American physician knows about as much about nutrition as his receptionist, unless she happens to have had a weight problem. Then she probably knows more."

Nutrition is not given a very important part in the medical school curriculum. A few lectures on vitamins, the different food groups, special diets for people with ulcers and other medical diseases may be all that passes for instruction in nutrition. The message during these lectures is usually that a "well-balanced diet provides all the nutrients that we need." The probability of the average American obtaining that "well-balanced diet" is not discussed or even considered. But the theory is correct. For most people, a well-balanced diet would provide the nutrients needed. The problem is most of us don't eat that kind of diet.

Senator George McGovern states in the forward to the 1975 Senate Select Committee Report on Nutrition and Health, "Americans who can afford an adequate diet may not be getting one either, however, for rich and poor alike are tempted daily by a food system thriving to expand demand by tempting the palate with foods overloaded with fat, sugar, and salt, low in nutritive value, high in pleasure value. Our eating habits and the composition of our food have changed radically, so what is happening to the nation's nutritional health?

"We know that millions of Americans are literally sick with diet-related illnesses. Five out of ten leading causes of death in the United States have been connected to diet.

"And millions of Americans are failing to realize their full potential because they do not have a proper diet. A recent study estimates that billions of dollars in economic benefits (to say nothing of spiritual benefits) are lost nationally each year because of improper nutrition."

Another contributing factor to the nutritional misinformation may be that even when a medical school has a strong nutrition department, many times the department is financed heavily by some of the food-processing companies whose products may be contributing to some of the nutritional woes we are experiencing. Obviously, the processing of foods for shipping and storage is essential. We have long ago passed the time when each of us was able to raise our own food. The problem is not with the processing. The problem is we are misled into believing that processed foods are as good as the real thing. Sometimes they are, but most of the time they're not. The facts can help us protect ourselves. By having large processing companies financially helping the nutrition departments of important universities, there is a potential conflict of interest. For some, it may be hard to bite the hand that feeds them; for others, it may be impossible.

Senator McGovern goes on to say, "Medical schools have underemphasized nutrition, with the result that the typical physical examination does not involve thorough nutritional evaluation or counseling." The starkest evidence of medical neglect with regard to nutrition is the meals served to patients in hospitals. Doctors traditionally have relied on dieticians to do nutrition examinations and counseling. Unfortunately, dieticians are not nutritionists, and so patients are often fed the very same types of refined foods that made them sick in the first place.

Another problem contributing to the medical establishment's lack of interest in a nutritional disease such as hypoglycemia is that the focus of American medicine is on crisis intervention—treating when the patient is sick. There is little or no attention given to the prevention and maintenance of good health. A patient with a heart attack, stroke, arthritis, arteriosclerosis, or hypertension will receive dedicated attention, but go to your doctor and say, "I'm feeling great. What can I do to stay that way?" and you may die in the waiting room before you get an answer. Nutrition is vitally important in the prevention of disease and in maintaining the good health most of us enjoy.

Whatever the many reasons an otherwise-intelligent, well-meaning physician closes down a trap door in his mind at the suggestion of hypoglycemia, the fact is too many patients are turned off, turned away, or diverted to other treatments by doctors who say, "There is no such thing as hypoglycemia."

Senator McGovern ends his forward by stating, "The strength of the nation is based on the health of its people. We must realize that the simple act of choosing our diet, day after day, determines our personal health and well may affect the health of other nations. Americans eat on as they have at their peril."

Finding a Doctor

The title of this book implies that your doctor probably qualifies as an expert in many essential areas of medicine, but that he may for one reason or another avoid considering hypoglycemia as a cause of your problems. In seeking help, try your doctor, though. Give him a chance. If, however, you are met with resistance, you may wish to contact one of the following sources for a physician who will be more in tune with the treatment of hypoglycemia.

In this time of specialization and even micro-specialization, all physicians cannot know and do all things. If your doctor does not wish to consider hypoglycemia as the cause of your problems, you may be able to find someone who treats low blood sugar by calling your local medical society. In most large cities, medical societies maintain a referral service, listing their member doctors with their specialties and interests.

If your own physician and the local medical society have been of no help in your quest to find a doctor willing to consider hypoglycemia, you may be able to obtain information from the following professional organizations made up of nutritionally minded physicians.

**ATKINS CENTER FOR
COMPLIMENTARY MEDICINE**
152 East 55th Street
New York, NY 10022

THE INSTITUTE FOR THE STUDY
OF OPTIMAL NUTRITION
2546 Regis Drive
Davis, CA 95616

ALACER CORPORATION
14 Morgan
Irvine, CA 92718

This is a commercial organization that is involved in the sale of many nutritional supplements. They have compiled a booklet listing nutritionally oriented physicians throughout the United States and will send it on request. There is a 50¢ handling charge.

After you have written to one of the above organizations and have received a list of referrals, it is best to then call the physician's office to make certain that he is familiar with the problem that you wish to have investigated. The organizations are in no way responsible for the proficiency of the doctors on their referral lists, but they do appreciate hearing positive or negative experiences that you might have had with the physicians on their list.

Chapter Four

What Is Hypoglycemia?

Our bodies are marvelous, miraculous machines with exquisite regulating mechanisms. In addition to maintaining heart rate, blood pressure, and respiratory rate, our bodies also maintain innumerable chemical levels in our blood. But when there is too much or too little of a certain substance, some health problems may develop. Too much sugar may cause diabetes, too much of the wrong kind of fat may contribute to arteriosclerosis, and too little potassium may cause heart problems. Hypo (low) glycemia (blood sugar) occurs when the body can no longer regulate the amount of sugar in the blood, which in turn causes the sugar level to fall to lower than an optimum level, or for it to fall too quickly.

When a person's blood has too little sugar in it to sustain bodily functions, several symptoms arise. Some of the symptoms are directly caused by the low level of sugar and can be relieved immediately by eating. When a patient has a history of these symptoms that were relieved by eating, there is a good chance that the person has hypoglycemia.

The first of these symptoms is confusion and the inability to think straight or to make up one's mind. One patient who was suffering from hypoglycemia went too long without eating and in an attempt to find some food went into about four restaurants, but he walked out of each one as quickly as he had walked in. He complained that each of the restaurants was either too dirty or too crowded, that the menus were too limited, that the tables were awkwardly placed, or that he didn't like the look of the customers. When he finally decided that his problem was his inability to make up his mind because his blood sugar was so low, he decided to force himself to eat in the next available restaurant. After he ate, he immediately felt better and thought more clearly.

The second symptom is hunger, caused by a drop in the blood sugar. Usually, the hunger is associated with a craving for something sweet, although some people crave starchy foods, which within the body are chemically the same as sweets, and some people crave alcohol.

The third symptom is tremulousness. As a young physician who was unaware of the importance of nutrition, I often skipped breakfast in favor of an ever-brewing pot of coffee in the doctor's lounge in the hospital where I worked. In addition to several cups of black coffee, I ate one or two doughnuts out of the carton supplied by myself or other equally uninformed physicians. This caffeine and sugar marathon started at 8 A.M. By around 11 A.M., I had such tremors that I often experienced difficulty signing my name. The tremors promptly disappeared after I ate lunch. Several years later, when I became interested in nutrition, I began to realize the stress I was putting myself under with my daily coffee and donut routine.

The fourth symptom is weakness and fainting. This occurs when the blood sugar is too low to maintain consciousness. Fainting is not a common symptom but has been known to occur in a small percentage of people with hypoglycemia.

I would like to emphasize that the above symptoms are immediate physical responses to a lowered sugar level. The person experiencing these symptoms often clearly links them to a lack of food and feels better once he has eaten.

These symptoms may occur in anyone who has skipped a meal, and are not of great significance since they are temporary and quickly reversed.

The more debilitating symptoms of hypoglycemia, and the ones that usually bring a patient to the doctor's office in search of help, are longer-lasting and not immediately relieved by eating. One of the most common of these symptoms is fatigue. Over 90 percent of the people who have hypoglycemia suffer from this symptom. I saw a typical example of this symptom in an attractive 23-year-old woman who came to my office. She moved slower than one would expect, and although she had paid some attention to her grooming, it was obvious that she did not pay close attention to it. She complained of being tired all the time and looked fatigued. Until three months prior to her visit, she had had a fairly interesting and responsible job as an executive secretary. As her work fell off during the year and as her fatigue increased, she was unable to maintain her usual proficiency. She noted, "It doesn't make any difference how much sleep I get. I am as tired after ten hours of sleep as I am after five."

Another common symptom is irritability, which makes being around a person with hypoglycemia trying and difficult and has led to problems within many marriages. The irritability may take the form of verbal abuse or may manifest itself in a physical action such as throwing a dish across a room. The slightest stimulus may trigger a rage. Patients who have experienced this type of almost uncontrollable irritability often describe the same strange sensation following the episode. "Physically, I felt much better, as if my body were relieved, but emotionally I felt terrible because I recognized my behavior was uncalled for." Other symptoms may develop when a person does not express the rage in a direct, open manner. Many people will hold their feelings inside. Their feelings of rage may manifest themselves in depression and withdrawal, or sometimes in other physical symptoms, such as an irritable colon, back pain, stomach pains, and headaches. I do not mean to imply that all psychiatric disorders and physical complaints in a person with hypoglycemia are the result of turned-in rage, but this turned-in rage may be an explanation for some of the physical complaints often seen in persons with hypoglycemia.

Another explanation for these complaints may be found in the chemical relationship between food and emotions. For example, interesting investigative work is being done in an attempt to unravel the connection between certain chemicals called neuro-transmitters and depression. Neuro transmitters are responsible for the movement of a nervous impulse from one cell to another. I believe that there is not only a connection between neuro-transmitters and the state of depression, but that there is also a relationship between neuro-transmitters and foods.

Besides this direct connection between sugar, neuro-transmitters, and depression, hypoglycemia itself undoubtedly has a more indirect psychological effect on the person who has had it and been untreated for many years. Months or years in which one feels tired, irritable, unable to think clearly or to start or accomplish tasks, resulting in interrupted and disorganized interpersonal relationships is clearly sufficient cause for depression and low self-esteem.

The case of Betty W. illustrates this point very well. Betty W., who was a 34-year-old married woman when she first saw me, noted that shortly after the birth of her first child, who was eight years old at the time, she became irritable and depressed. She had been married for only a year when her child was born, and although Betty cared for her husband and he for her very much, she was concerned that the birth of their first child at a time when they were both struggling financially was going to be too much of a burden. Although her husband reassured her frequently that he wanted the child, she remained doubtful. When she was depressed and irritable following the birth of the child, at first everyone advised her that this would pass and that it was common.

Several months went by, however, and since she was becoming more depressed rather than less, her husband finally convinced her to see a psychiatrist. By this time, she was doing very little of her household work and her child would have been neglected if it hadn't been for her mother, who came in every day to help. With the help of some antidepressants and psychotherapy, Betty became less depressed and was able to assume a little more of the responsibilities of the housework, but she continued to have extremely little energy. For years following the birth of her child, she continued to go to bed shortly after dinner, and she withdrew even more from her husband. Although he tried in vain for all those years to maintain good contact with her, he eventually gave up, and although they continued to live together, exchanging cross words, they shared only a house and a child, and had very little else in common. Her mother insisted that Betty be examined further, which led to the diagnosis of hypoglycemia. After four to five months of changed eating habits, people remarked that she was a "different person." She was seldom depressed, and her energy gradually improved to a point where she felt wonderful with only seven to eight hours of sleep a night. She was able to take care of her house and found herself cleaning closets and cupboards that hadn't been touched for years. The only thing that didn't improve was her relationship with her husband. He saw the difference in his wife, but remained somewhat distrustful, and unsure it would last. This was understandable; for years, they had grown apart. After I explained this situation to both of them, I suggested they try marriage counseling and they agreed, for neither of them wanted to end the relationship.

At the present, they are still being counseled, and although their relationship has improved, it is difficult to say whether the scars caused by Betty's illness will be erased sufficiently for them to continue to be together. One can't help but wonder what a different life the entire family would have had if Betty had been treated promptly.

So far, I have mentioned only a few of the devastating and sometimes crippling symptoms of hypoglycemia. A complete list was compiled by Dr. S. Gyland, a practicing physician and himself a hypoglycemia sufferer. After he had treated more than 600 patients for the disease, he compiled the following list of symptoms, along with their frequency.

Experienced by over 90 percent of hypoglycemics:
 Nervousness
Experienced by over 80 percent:
 Irritability
 Exhaustion, unexplained tiredness
 Faintness
 Dizziness
 Tremors
 Cold sweats
 Weak spells
Experienced by over 70 percent:
 Depression
 Vertigo
 Drowsiness
 Headaches
Experienced by over 60 percent:
 Digestive disturbances
 Forgetfulness
 Insomnia
 Constant worrying
 Anxieties
Experienced by over 50 percent:
 Obesity
 Mental confusion
 Palpitations
 Muscle pain
 Indecisiveness
 Numbness

Experienced by over 40 percent:
    Asthma
    Unsocial, asocial, or antisocial behavior
    Crying spells
    Lack of sex drive
    Allergies and respiratory problems
    Lack of coordination
    Leg cramps
    Lack of concentration
    Blurred vision
    Twitching and jerking muscles
Experienced by over 30 percent:
    Itching and crawling sensations on the skin
    Gasping for breath
    Smothering spells
    Staggering
    Sighing and yawning
Experienced by over 20 percent:
    Impotency (males)
    Night terrors
    Arthritis
    Phobias
    Fears
    Skin conditions
    Suicidal impulses
Experienced by over 10 percent:
    Nervous breakdowns
Experienced by over 2 percent:
    Convulsions

The symptoms, both the physical and the psychological, have many causes. These may be broken down as follows:

1. Related to the direct lack of nutrients. This may cause such symptoms as temporary confusion, acute fatigue, and tremors.

2. The probable effect on the neuro-transmitters of the high intake of sugar. This is a presumed cause for a symptom

such as depression. Much more investigation will have to be done before this is completely understood or validated.

3. The effect of the regulatory changes that the body has to go through in order to correct the low blood sugar. When one's blood sugar drops too suddenly or to a level that is too low to maintain body functions satisfactorily, a tremendous stress is put on the body. Adrenaline is released, which in turn causes the release of stored carbohydrates. Anyone who has ever had an injection of Adrenalin with novocaine by a dentist knows the uncomfortable sensation of a speeding heart and the accompanying sensation of fear caused by the increased amount of adrenaline in the system. In a person with hypoglycemia, adrenaline may be released frequently throughout the day. It is the adrenaline that accounts for some of the anxieties, as well as for some of the tremors and general feeling of "nervousness" so often experienced by hypoglycemics. Adrenaline also is the hormone that is released when we have to fight an opponent or to run from one. In a hypoglycemic, who is neither fighting nor running, the increased amounts of adrenaline easily contribute to the feeling of irritability that makes the person look for a fight.

Chapter Five

Making the Diagnosis

If you consume sugar (not only table sugar but sugar in packaged and canned foods), fruit, milk, and the like, and you do not feel 100% perfect, then try the following;

For two weeks eat only protein (fish, fowl, soy, nuts, and seeds) and vegetables, and snack on these in between meals, if needed. Your symptoms of dis-ease will probably disappear. This is a very simple and effective way of diagnosing reactive hypoglycemia. However, if you feel the need for a laboratory test, then you should go for a glucose tolerance test.

On arrival at the laboratory, a vial of blood is drawn and the subject is given a measured amount of glucose dissolved in liquid. Blood samples should then be drawn $1/2$ hour, 1, 2, $3\,1/2$, 4, and 5 hours after the patient has the drink. The first $1/2$-hour specimen is not routinely done in some laboratories and this is unfortunate since it is sometimes a very important specimen.

The blood samples are then examined for their actual sugar content. In the metric system, a cubic centimeter (cc) is a measure of volume. A milligram (mg), $1/1,000$ of a gram, is a measure of weight. The amount of sugar in the blood is expressed in terms of the weight of the sugar (mg) in the specific volume (cc) of blood. For example, during the so-called fast, a normal reading is usually between 80 and 100 mg of sugar for every 100 cc of blood, expressed as 80 to 100 mg percent.

By giving many people a five-hour glucose tolerance test, normal values have been obtained. A normal glucose tolerance curve is shown in Figure 1, it plots the amount of sugar in 100 cc of blood, against the time: fasting, $\frac{1}{2}$ hour, 1 hour, 2 hours, 3 hours, 4 hours, and 5 hours after the glucose. All of the readings need not fall exactly into the normal range for a person to be normal, but there are several critical factors to be considered: (1) The fasting level should be within the normal range. (2) Within the first hour, the blood sugar should raise a minimum of half more than the fasting level. Although the graph shows the high level of sugar at 1 hour, it is perfectly normal to have this level at the $\frac{1}{2}$-hour reading, with a return to the fasting level at the end of the hour. As stated before, the $\frac{1}{2}$-hour specimen is sometimes very important in determining whether or not there has been a rise in blood sugar level. (3) At the second hour, the blood sugar should return to within a short range of the fasting level. (4) All blood specimens from the second hour through the sixth hour should remain close to the fasting levels.

A person is diagnosed as having hypoglycemia when there are more than normal variations in the glucose tolerance curve. It is in the interpretation of the test where there is considerable difference of opinion. I'm not talking about those physicians who don't believe in hypoglycemia, because obviously they should never order a 5-hour glucose tolerance test in the first place.

Most laboratory tests furnish information that must be used in conjunction with other findings, in order to arrive at a proper interpretation. For the most part physicians interpreting laboratory tests want to see a consistency between the patient's symptoms and the abnormal test results, yet, more often than not, the results of the glucose tolerance test are inter-

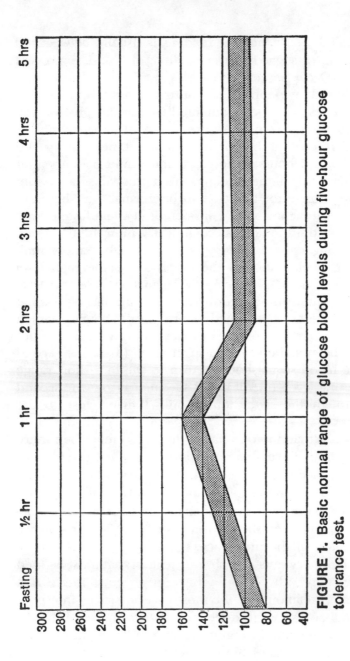

FIGURE 1. Basic normal range of glucose blood levels during five-hour glucose tolerance test.

preted on the basis of only one criteria: did the blood sugar level fall below a specified level? The level is arbitrarily set at 50 mg percent by some physicians. If the physician looks only for a drop below 50 mg percent, he will miss diagnosing 95 percent of the people with treatable hypoglycemia. Remember, in making a laboratory diagnosis of hypoglycemia, it is not only necessary to conduct the test properly but to interpret the results properly.

Dr. Seale Harris, the physician who first described hypoglycemia, found that while his hypoglycemia patients were having symptoms, their blood sugar level was below 60 mg percent. For many years, this sole criterion was used to make the laboratory diagnosis of hypoglycemia, and a drop below a specified blood sugar level frequently is still the one and only bit of information used to make a diagnosis. The only difference is, throughout the years, the level has been getting lower and lower. Such a changing level is entirely predictable as physicians try to "prove" that hypoglycemia doesn't exist. Consistent with the effort of the medical establishment to prove that hypoglycemia is nonexistent, a study was published that showed that if normal men fasted for several days their blood sugars would reach 30 mg percent during a glucose tolerance test. The inference is that a blood sugar level had to drop to 30 mg before a diagnosis of hypoglycemia should be made. Such a conclusion would be correct if we usually were fasting, but since the fasting state is the exception, certainly laboratory results based on a fast are the exception and do not apply to our usual nourished state, even a generally poor nourished state.

The biggest problem in basing the diagnosis on some figures on a piece of paper is that a fundamental rule of medicine is violated. The rule is "Treat the patient not the laboratory results." There are many patients who have been through the unpleasantness of the five-hour glucose tolerance test without ever being questioned about their reactions during the test. But because the figures failed to show a level below the 60 or 50 or 40 mg percent, whatever absolute figures might be in vogue at the time, the patient was told, "You don't have hypoglycemia."

One young woman with a "normal test" felt so faint throughout the test and had such violent headaches that she could barely move. A middle-aged man experienced many symptoms of depression, anxiety, and backaches throughout the test. Yet these patients were told that their tests were normal. Of course, some of these symptoms may have been caused by a multitude of other problems, but the subject's reactions must be considered in reaching a diagnosis. Ignoring the patient always reminds me of a cartoon I saw of a man lying in a hospital bed bandaged from head to foot. The physician standing by him states, "Your tests are all normal. You can go home now." As physicians, we sometimes forget that the laboratory is only an aid and an adjunct to diagnosis, not the final word.

One of the first doctors to realize that the laboratory criteria were not enough to diagnose hypoglycemia was Dr. H. Saltzer. This astute physician recognized that many of his patients had definite symptoms during the five-hour glucose tolerance test, even though their blood sugar level did not fall below the then-accented level necessary to make the diagnosis. After studying these patients, Dr. Saltzer concluded that many patients might develop symptoms of hypoglycemia even though their blood sugar levels were above what was described as normal.

Just as our heart rates, blood pressures, temperatures, cholesterol levels, sodium levels, and other measurable figures vary from individual to individual, so, too, our body chemistries vary. Dr. Saltzer in his article on relative hypoglycemia (*Journal of the National Medical Association,* January, 1966) described criteria for laboratory diagnosis of hypoglycemia that allow for individual differences in biochemistry. In essence, he reasoned that each of us has our own normal blood sugar level, which is the fasting level, or the level of the blood sugar after we have had no food for several hours. He found that a drop below that level could result in symptoms of hypoglycemia. He also made another interesting observation, namely, that when the blood sugar level dropped rapidly from one hour to the next, hypoglycemic symptoms might also appear. Dr. Saltzer described these conditions as relative hypoglycemia. This means that during the five-hour test, a blood sugar sample is low relative to the fasting or normal blood sugar for the person being tested. It is the group of relative hypoglycemic patients that are so often misdiagnosed as normal.

Specifically, Dr. Saltzer said that a person has relative hypoglycemia if at any time during the glucose tolerance test (1) the blood sugar falls 20 mg percent below the fasting level and if at that particular level the person is experiencing symptoms; or (2) if there is a drop of 50 mg percent or more within one hour and the person is experiencing symptoms. These symptoms may be any of a number of hypoglycemic symptoms such as weakness, sleepiness, tremors, hunger, anxiety, rapid pulse, sweating, headaches, depression, or general nervousness. See Figures 2 and 3.

There are two other laboratory results that suggest hypoglycemia: a flat curve or a sawtooth curve. The former exists when the blood sugar fails to reach a minimum $1/2$ times greater than the fasting value within the first hour after drinking the glucose. See Figure 4. The sawtooth curve exists when the blood sugar level peaks a second time after the initial rise within the first hour. See Figure 5.

Thus, it becomes evident that there are several criteria that should be used before a laboratory diagnosis of hypoglycemia can be made. (1) The blood sugar should fall below a specified level such as 50 mg percent in any specimen taken during the glucose tolerance test. This condition usually indicates that the patient has reactive hypoglycemia. See Figure 6. If the fasting level is very low, the patient may have fasting hypoglycemia. This condition should be investigated to determine whether the person has a possible enlargement or tumors of the pancreas. In terms of the total number of people with hypoglycemic conditions, enlargement or tumors of the pancreas are *very rare*. *(2) A fall in the blood sugar level of 20 mg percent or more below the fasting level, accompanied by symptoms. (3) A fall in the blood sugar level of 50 percent or more within any hour, accompanied by symptoms. (4) A flat curve. (5) A sawtooth curve.*

During a glucose tolerance test, the patient ideally should be watched for reactions and extra blood samples should be drawn during the reactions. Other variations in the testing, such as $1/2$-hour samples throughout instead of hourly samples, can also be done. Of course, from the standpoint of diagnosis, the more samples the better. From the standpoint of the patient's punctured arm and punctured purse, too many tests may not be desirable. For most people who have hypoglycemia, a laboratory test conducted in the routine manner with the fasting $1/2$-hour, 1-, 2-, 3-, $31/2$, 4-, and 5-hour samples will be sufficient to make a diagnosis. I have seen a few tests in which frequent readings were done, showing a drop between the hours with a return to the acceptable level within the hour. Without the extra $1/2$-hour samples, these abnormal glucose tolerance tests would have appeared normal. Taking a specimen after $31/2$ hours usually reveals abnormalities that would have been missed as well. You must request this specimen since it is not usually done.

In the absence of a trained technician who can watch for symptoms and draw extra samples, the person taking the test should be asked to keep a diary of any reactions experienced during the five hours. At times, patients may be instructed to request that an extra blood sample be drawn if obvious symptoms such as rapid pulse, sweating, sudden weakness, or loss of color develop at least 15 minutes before the next blood sample is to be drawn.

Because the blood sugar level may drop and then rapidly

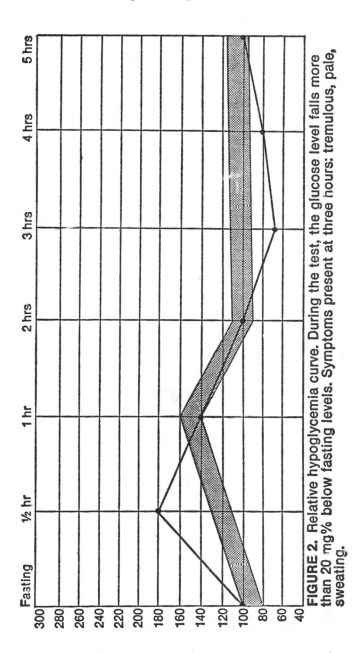

FIGURE 2. Relative hypoglycemia curve. During the test, the glucose level falls more than 20 mg% below fasting levels. Symptoms present at three hours: tremulous, pale, sweating.

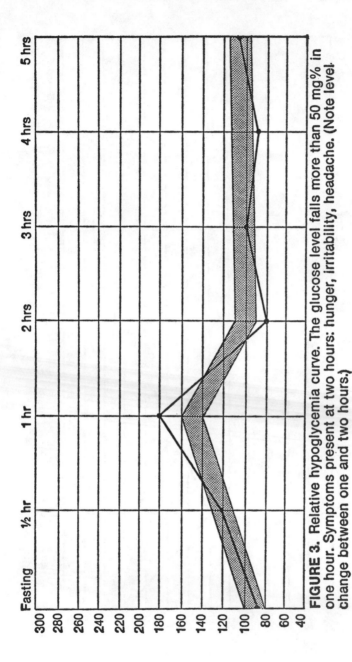

FIGURE 3. Relative hypoglycemia curve. The glucose level falls more than 50 mg% in one hour. Symptoms present at two hours: hunger, irritability, headache. (Note level change between one and two hours.)

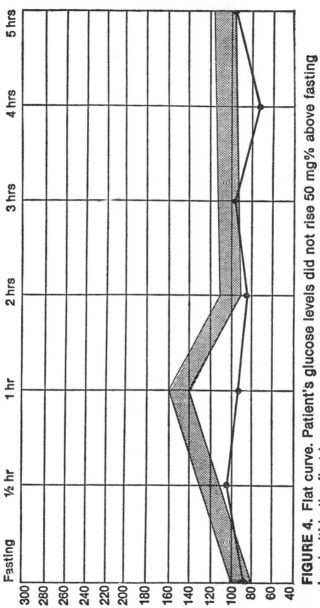

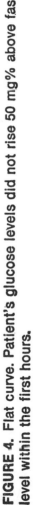

FIGURE 4. Flat curve. Patient's glucose levels did not rise 50 mg% above fasting level within the first hours.

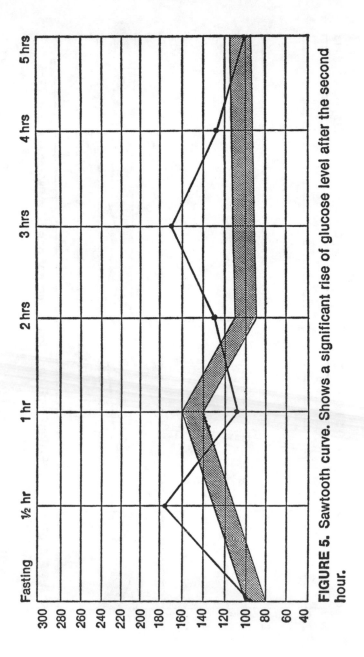

FIGURE 5. Sawtooth curve. Shows a significant rise of glucose level after the second hour.

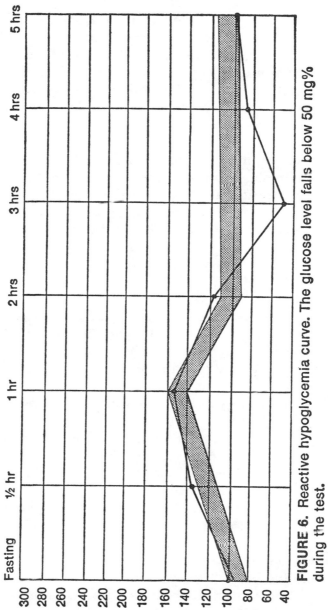

FIGURE 6. Reactive hypoglycemia curve. The glucose level falls below 50 mg% during the test.

correct itself during the test, there is some justification in treating the person for hypoglycemia when the history is strongly suggestive and the symptoms present during the test, even if the laboratory results are normal. Such a situation arises only rarely, but obviously it is important for people who might otherwise have gone untreated. In the very few instances when I have treated these people, the results often justified the decision.

There are many other advantages to the glucose tolerance test in addition to its being an aid in diagnosis. If the laboratory can show that a patient's test results are abnormal, the patient usually will muster up the discipline needed to follow a prescribed diet. Without laboratory proof, the determination to stay on the diet usually fades with the rationalization "I don't really know if this diet is important or not."

The glucose tolerance test is also helpful in that it indicates whether further testing should be done to determine if there may be a serious physical cause for the hypoglycemia, such as a rare tumor of the pancreas. An organic cause for hypoglycemia should be thought of if the fasting specimen or any of the other specimens drop to a very low level. Although tumors are very rarely the cause of hypoglycemia, they must be ruled out in the above-mentioned cases.

Another advantage of the glucose tolerance test is that it may help in the determination of certain specifics of the diet, such as when the patient should have a snack. The test may also give a clue as to the expected treatment time since flat curves and sawtooth curves may indicate that a longer period of treatment will be required before there will be any response.

The important question asked by many people who undergo the test is "How serious is my condition?" The glucose tolerance test may indicate the need for further studies, especially if the patient has fasting hypoglycemia, but beyond that, the severity of the symptoms is not correlated to the particular configuration of the test results. I have seen test results that were so low that most physicians would agree that hypoglycemia existed, yet the symptoms were minimal. As an example, I remember a very beautiful actress who consulted me because she was feeling "run down." Her glucose tolerance test showed a third-hour specimen of 38 mg percent, indicating obvious hypoglycemia. Yet her career has kept her traveling and working almost constantly, so she has failed to follow up these findings. Although symptoms are definitely present, her determination and personality have allowed her to continue to function on her normal level. On the other hand, there are patients whose glucose tolerance results show minimal changes but who exhibit maximum symptoms that improve once the patient has the proper treatment. The severity of the illness cannot be predicted by the test results.

If there is anything nice about hypoglycemia, it is that once the condition is properly diagnosed, the treatment in most instances is simple and the results are predictable. As a physician, it is particularly gratifying to be able to see people start to enjoy life simply by getting them to pay attention to the basics of good nutrition, which is what the treatment of hypoglycemia is all about.

Chapter Six

The Treatment

The logical approach to the treatment of low blood sugar would seem to be to eat more sugar. But logic only works if the premises are correct. Anyone who advises a person with hypoglycemia to eat more sugar, is not working with the correct premise. Low blood sugar is not caused by a lack of sugar in the diet. It is caused by the failure of the body's sugar-regulating mechanism, which results in a lowered sugar level in the blood after the person has eaten sugar. The obvious treatment then would be to not eat sugar. However, in treating the condition, this advice is too vague and is usually not sufficient to correct it. There are three dietary rules I advise my patients to follow: (1) watch what you eat, (2) how much you eat, and (3) when you eat.

What You Eat

There are three basic food groups: carbohydrates, proteins, and fats. Proper amounts of these foodstuffs are necessary for optimum health, although not everyone has the same requirements for each food group. A person who has hypoglycemia should have absolutely no refined carbohy-

drates, but may have complex carbohydrates (e.g., gr...
Refined carbohydrates are the lifeless processed starches
and sugars. The use of the word *sugars* is confusing. At one
time, it is used as a description for all carbohydrates. At
other times, it is used to designate that stuff we find on our
tables and add to our foods, whether it is white, brown,
multicolored, or powdered.

When a natural fruit such as a beet is treated so that the
carbohydrates are extracted, the end product is table sugar,
or a refined carbohydrate. Another refined carbohydrate is
white flour. Even small amounts of refined carbohydrates
can set in motion an abnormal reaction in some hypoglycemic patients.

Refined carbohydrates are everywhere. A person who is
being treated for hypoglycemia must read labels. Refined
sugar is added to so many foods that a little here and there
may add up to more than can be handled. Sugar is found
in unlikely places such as canned baby foods, canned soups,
vegetables, sauces, ketchup, and salad dressings. Although
all packaged foods must be labeled, manufacturers now use
synonyms for sugar, such as dextrose, sucrose, glucose, or
natural sweetener. There are many different carbohydrates
(sugars), but whenever they are concentrated and used as
sweeteners, they should be avoided. For hypoglycemics, it is
the amount, or the concentration, of the carbohydrate that
leads to the trouble, so all refined carbohydrates should be
avoided since they are really the troublemaking ones.

Some fruits, though very nutritious, are too high in carbohydrates to be tolerated by some persons with hypoglycemia. The fresh fruits with highly concentrated amounts
of natural sugar are bananas, apples, grapes, mangoes, and
all dried fruit. Although these are nutritious, the hypoglycemic should use them sparingly and only after the initial
treatment is over.

Sometimes there seems to be a great disagreement among
doctors who treat hypoglycemia. In reality, the disagreements

are over what constitutes the proper amount of carbohydrates. One physician may advise no milk because of the milk
sugar, or lactose. Another may advise staying away from certain fruits and vegetables that another physician may allow.
The controversy exists because there is no one diet that can
be effective for 100 percent of those who need it. We all vary
in our biochemical make-up, and what may be the correct
amount of carbohydrates for one person may be too much
for another. In practice, there is no way to determine what
an individual needs. The diet that is recommended in this
book has been shown through experience to benefit most
people who use it. If the diet is basically successful, variations
can be tried later on to truly personalize it. Since there will
be a small group on either side of the norm, one requiring
more carbohydrates, the other less, adjustments may have to
be made during the clinical course of treatment.

Refined carbohydrates and concentrated natural carbohydrates are not the only culprit for a person with hypoglycemia. Caffeine is another one. Even a schoolchild knows that
caffeine is an ingredient in coffee, but it is also found in
many teas, over-the-counter medications designed to ease
pain or fight drowsiness, and as an additive in many colas.
Again, you *must* read labels. Avoid caffeine. The problem
with caffeine is that it causes the release of sugar that has
been stored in the body. Once this sugar gets into the bloodstream, it is handled in the same maladaptive way as if it
came from ice cream.

Good-quality carbohydrates, on the other hand, are essential, so essential that our miracle machine is able to convert
some of the protein we eat into carbohydrates if needed.
While this is an expensive way to get carbohydrates, it may
be acceptable in the beginning of treatment, for when proteins are converted into carbohydrates under proper circumstances, it happens at a *slow* rate that does not upset or
challenge the sugar mechanism. It is large concentrations of
sugar that cannot be handled, so that the slow conversion of

some of the protein to sugar may be ideal in the beginning of treatment. Alcohol inhibits this conversion, thus resulting in a very low level of carbohydrates in those people who are depending on the conversion of the protein into the carbohydrates. Other alcoholic beverages such as wines and liqueurs contain large amounts of sugar. All alcoholic beverages should be avoided.

There are differences of opinion among some physicians concerning the use of artificial sweeteners. For several reasons, I advise my patients to avoid them, especially in the early stages of treatment. Although I am not aware of any scientific work substantiating the hypothesis, I think there is a possibility that the sugar-regulating mechanism may be set into motion with the taste of something sweet. It is well-known that many digestive enzymes start finding their way into the digestive system at the first sensation of the taste of food. Years ago, some studies showed that in at least one case even taste wasn't necessary. As the person smelled cooking bacon, the enzymes that would be necessary to break down that bacon were already being emptied into the stomach. Likewise, a sweet taste may cause the release of insulin.

Another reason to avoid artificial sweeteners is that they are artificial. Each day, we are subjected to so many environmental insults over which we have little control, when we have a free choice, why add other chemicals that are potentially harmful?

Yet another reason to avoid sweeteners is that the sweet taste, which many feel they cannot live without, is an acquired taste. After successful treatment, any food with added sugar usually has an undesirable sweetness. When the person who has been treated finds that his old sugar standbys no longer have the pleasurable sensation they once had, it is then much easier to stay on a diet that eliminates refined carbohydrates. On the other hand, if the person has been eating some type of sweetener, there is no change of taste, and going back to the usual sugar foods is very easy. Avoiding the extra sweetened foods during the period of treatment results in a refinement of taste that allows the need for sweets to be satisfied by natural foods such as fruits.

Some people mention honey as a natural sweetener, and it is. But it is too concentrated for hypoglycemics. Do without sweeteners. Be good to yourself. Learn what food tastes like. Don't add sweeteners of any kind.

Tobacco also has been found to lower the blood sugar and should be avoided. In my own practice, I usually handle this topic separately. In some instances, the added advice to stop smoking is too drastic and creates so much stress that the overall effect is that the patient ignores all advice, including the dietary. If I am questioned about tobacco when the treatment begins, I always advise that the patient stop smoking if possible. If I am not questioned, I wait until a later date when the patient usually mentions that he doesn't feel particularly well when smoking. At this time, I confirm the observation and recommend that it would be easier to stop or reduce smoking now than it would have been earlier in the treatment.

A word of caution should be included about *marijuana*. Anyone who uses this drug is familiar with the "munchies," an intense desire to eat. The desire for sweet foods may be particularly strong. On marijuana, there is heightened sensitivity, especially for food, where so many senses are stimulated—sight, taste, feel—that it becomes obvious that marijuana can be disastrous for anyone trying to *control* what he eats and especially how much he eats.

How Much You Eat

In the treatment of hypoglycemia, paying attention to what you eat is not enough. How much you eat is also very important. Meals must be small. Small is a frustrating term for anyone who wants to be precise, but an exact amount cannot be determined. Small is a relative term and means different things to different people. A small amount for a 200-pound football player is not a small amount for a 105-pound secretary. In determining what is a small amount, there are two rules: (1) Eat enough so that you are not hungry, (2) do not eat enough to feel stuffed. The object is to hold down the amount of available food that can or could be converted to sugar. If you have eaten a large amount of food, there is the possibility that an oversupply of sugar will exist as part of the food is turned into sugar.

When You Eat

The third important dietary rule concerns when you eat. A person who begins treatment must "eat by the clock, not by the stomach." The dietary program is designed to prevent a drop in blood sugar. The glucose tolerance test is very helpful in deciding the frequency of the snacks. A snack should be taken at a time *prior* to the drop of the sugar level, as shown in the person's glucose tolerance curve. For example, if the glucose tolerance curve revealed a low level at the third hour of the test, then the advice would be to snack every two hours between meals and until bedtime. If there was a low level the fifth hour, the advice would be to snack every four hours, and so on. Snacking every few hours or so isn't too difficult, but sometimes there is a drop the first hour or even the second hour. In some of these cases, I have not seen satisfactory improvement until snacks were taken at a frequency to prevent the drop in sugar. In those instances, patients sometimes do not eat regular meals but find themselves constantly snacking. Fortunately, the need for such frequent snacks is rare.

SUMMARY: The dietary plan is as follows:
   1. Watch what you eat. Avoid *all* processed carbohy-

drates. Eat only complex carbohydrates and moderate amounts of protein and fats.
2. Watch how much you eat. Eat frequent small meals, enough to prevent hunger, but not enough to be stuffed.
3. Watch when you eat. Eat meals and snacks by the clock to avoid the drop in blood sugar.

I suggest the following for a hypoglycemic diet:

ALLOWABLE FOODS

Meats—any unprocessed fish, fowl, or other animal or vegetable protein
Liquids—vegetable juices, herbal teas, decaffeinated coffee, plain soda, all mineral waters or other bottled waters, milk
Vegetables—preferably fresh, steamed, or raw

Asparagus	Olives
Bean sprouts	Artichokes
Broccoli	Beets
Cabbage	Brussel sprouts
Cauliflower	Carrots
Celery	Chives
Cucumber	Eggplant
Lettuce	Okra
Mushrooms	Onions
Sauerkraut	Parsley
Spinach	Peppers
Squash	Pimento
String beans	Pumpkin
Tomatoes	Turnips
Avocados	Tomato puree

Fruits—any fresh and raw (use sparingly)

Cantaloupe	Boysenberries
Rhubarb	Coconut
Strawberries	Cranberries
Grapefruit	Papayas
Melons	Peaches
Lemons/Limes	Tangerines
Watermelon	

Nuts and Seeds—any (preferably raw)
Dairy—any dairy product including yogurt, plain only
Grains—any whole grains
Bread—whole-grain bread only

FOODS TO AVOID

Any foods containing sugar, white flour, white rice, artificial sweeteners, honey, caffeine, alcohol, or vinegar.

RESTRICTIONS

1. Fruits—only after the initial treatment is over and then no more than two servings daily
2. Milk—a limit of two eight-ounce glasses daily
3. Bread—a limit to one piece of yeast-free whole-grain bread daily

A SAMPLE DIET

Breakfast

Choose from eggs, cheese, meat, fish, or fowl. Grains—any whole grain or four- or seven-grain hot cereal. Beverage—any allowable beverage.

Lunch and Dinner

Choose from meat, fish, or fowl. Allowable vegetable and/or salad. Fruit if allowed.

Snacks

Choose from small portions of meat, dairy products, nuts, or seeds. Two tablespoons of flavored liquid protein is usually a sufficient nutrient for a snack. This is particularly useful for people who are unable to get to a food source and also for those who would gain weight by eating nuts, dairy products, and meats frequently throughout the day.

A WORD OF CAUTION

The above diet is a satisfactory treatment diet for most people with hypoglycemia. Some may require more complex carbohydrates, some less. The treatment diet is usually followed for a minimum of four months, at which time a gradually expanded diet is tried to provide more interest and more nutrients.

Grains and dairy products present a special problem because of a high frequency of grain and dairy sensitivity. The use of complex carbohydrates (grains) is satisfactory for some but not for all. The individuality of response necessitates close self-observation.

ALLERGIES

Allergies and hypoglycemia seem to go hand in hand. There are arguments on both sides of the issue concerning which causes the other. For years, it has been known that allergies disappear during the treatment of hypoglycemia. On the other hand, there are some positive indications that strongly suggest the problem being treated is an allergy rather than hypoglycemia. When the symptoms disappear abruptly after the first four to seven days on the diet, and that improvement persists, I believe an allergy rather than hypoglycemia was responsible for the symptoms.

Other Considerations

Experiments have shown that it is advisable to have an especially high-quality breakfast (whole grains, eggs, etc.) as opposed to the usual low-quality carbohydrate breakfast. Normal subjects who ate a breakfast high in sugar demonstrated problems in sugar control throughout the day and with all of the following meals. Those who had a high-quality breakfast (see Vim and Vigor Diet, Chapter 15) had no problem controlling their sugar levels when they ate additional meals throughout the day. This finding has special significance for the person with low blood sugar, who should make an effort to have foods of high quality for breakfast.

In addition to recommending the proper diet, I give my patients supplements of yeast-free natural B vitamins. The best B supplement is a B Complex tablet that has at least 50 mg of all known natural B vitamins. This can be taken two or three times a day after meals. The B vitamins are very important in the chemical processes that are involved in the utilization of carbohydrates. A few patients I have seen did not improve until the B vitamins were added. In addition to the B vitamins, I usually order at least 1,000 mg of natural vitamin C and 400 units of natural vitamin E twice a day after meals, for general health.

Minerals are vital links in the metabolism of carbohydrates. Scientists have found that chromium and manganese are very important for proper glucose metabolism. Minerals are undoubtedly important for the maintenance of good health. Since the person who goes on a hypoglycemic diet usually increases the amount of proteins he consumes, it is advisable that he take a multi-mineral supplement, since proteins do increase the need for minerals. I usually use a chelated multi-mineral since the chelated form is supposed to be absorbed into the body easier than the non-chelated forms.

Dr. Paavo Airola has made a clear distinction in his book. *Hypoglycemia: A Better Approach* (Health Plus Publications, 1977) between the refined carbohydrates such as table sugar and the complex carbohydrates found in whole grains. He points out that people who have hypoglycemia are not able to tolerate refined carbohydrates, but do tolerate and improve when complex carbohydrates are used in the treatment. The addition of whole grains releases carbohydrates more slowly than the refined sugars. The complex carbohydrates have been shown to be useful in correcting the physical slump that commonly occurs during the first stage of treatment. The addition of the complex carbohydrates is a valuable contribution to the treatment of hypoglycemia in many patients.

J. Daniel Palm, Ph.D., writes in *Diet Away Your Stress, Tension, and Anxiety* of the value of fructose, or fruit sugar, in the treatment of hypoglycemia. Some people who have hypoglycemia are able to tolerate *small* amounts of fructose without having a hypoglycemic episode. In my experience, however, most patients react unfavorably to fructose. I limit its use to those who are unwilling to accept a diet without some sweets. Those who use fructose may never have the experience of discovering that sweetness is an acquired taste and one that can be unlearned. Although fructose is said to be safe for hypoglycemics because it is not supposed to trigger the sugar-controlling mechanism that results in the low blood sugar levels, in my experience, it is not always safe. I have seen some patients react to fructose with the usual hypoglycemic symptoms. In addition, fructose has been available in the refined form for only a few years. It is possible that if fructose were used over a number of years in the same quantities that other refined sugars have been used, we would soon see similar problems developing from the overconsumption of fructose. Fructose may have a part to play in the treatment of hypoglycemia, but it is only a very limited part and only in very few instances where compliance with the diet is otherwise impossible. If you must cheat, the best choice is the new liquid sweetener, Stevia Extract. You may also use granulated Sucanat, which is evaporated cane juice that has the nutrients retained. The author of the authorative newsletter "Naturally Well," Dr. Marcus Laux has observed that Sucanat doesn't jolt the blood sugar like refined sugar because it not only contains all the nutrients but also has a lower glycemic index than refined sugar.

Chapter Seven

What Can Be Expected

Disappointment is in store for those who start a diet and expect immediate results. It is easy to understand that when one gives up his favorite sugary foods and has to fight a craving, a reward is expected. The reward of better health does come, but not immediately.

When I first started working with patients with hypoglycemia, some of them complained about feeling bad when they started the diet. I assumed the program was incorrect and stopped it. Since then, I have learned to expect an initial difficult period for the patients and warn them about it and encourage them throughout it.

Three fairly distinct stages of recovery have been observed, each with its own characteristics. In each stage, patients tend to react in the same manner. Because the reaction may be discouraging to the patient, the physician is in a position to be of help as a teacher and guide. The patient's family may also be an effective therapeutic force if the physician has informed them what to expect. By informing them, family members or friends can help the patient on a day-to-day basis through some of the more demanding times during the treatment. Many individuals treated for hypoglycemia have the faith to continue the treatment and follow instructions if they are informed about what to expect and if methods for handling each stage are suggested to them.

The duration of each stage is usually three to five weeks and should be approximately the same for stages 1, 2, and 3. Variations do exist, and I have seen a few individuals go through a stage every week while others go through one every 2½ months. But by far, in the greatest number of cases, the stages last from three to five weeks.

First Stage

The first stage is the most difficult both psychologically and physically. This is the time when the patient expects the most and gets the least. There are two main characteristics of this stage: (1) The patient usually feels worse, for example, more fatigued and depressed. (2) There is a tremendous craving for sugar. Even though everyone is warned before starting this diet that he can expect to feel worse, many people don't understand what this means until they experience it. Many times, I have received a telephone call one to two weeks after a patient has started the diet that sounds as if it's the same recording playing over and over.

"Hello, Doctor, this is Mr. Elmore."

"Yes, Mr. Elmore?"

"I feel terrible."

"Hm."

"I'm weaker than I was before I started the diet."

"When did you start?"

"About one week ago."

"Yes, anything else?"

"I feel faint throughout the day. My work is not getting done. All I do at home is lie around and feel more depressed than I did before I started the diet. Some mornings, I feel I can't even get out of bed."

"Mr. Elmore, do you remember I told you that you would most likely feel worse during the first three to five weeks?"

Then comes the line that I've heard over and over.

"Yes, I know you said I might feel bad, but I didn't think that you meant this bad."

These symptoms are probably a result of not having enough good-quality carbohydrates in the diet. If the symptoms are minimal, the patient is encouraged to stay on the low-carbohydrate diet. However, if these symptoms become debilitating, as in the above case, more carbohydrates are added in the form of two to three small servings of allowable fruit a day, instead of the one that had been allowed. Perhaps I might add one or two extra slices of whole-grain bread a day to supply more carbohydrates or two cups of cooked whole grains. This may be given in the form of a hot four- or seven-grain cereal of brown rice, millet, barley, oats, buckwheat, or groats. Generally, the symptoms during the first stage are directly proportionate to the amount of sugar the person has been eating. If a nutritional evaluation indicates that the person has been eating a great amount of sugar, such as 20 to 100 teaspoons per day, which is not at all uncommon, I often start the diet with the addition of two cups of cooked whole grains daily, which seems to modify the extreme fatigue that is otherwise to be expected. By very carefully adding extra high-quality carbohydrates, such as more walnuts and cashews, some of the more difficult symptoms are usually modified. About the only comfort derived from feeling so terrible during the first stage is that it was anticipated and does indicate that changes are taking place. If this stage occurs as anticipated, there is a likelihood that the expected improvement will also follow.

The other characteristic of the first stage is the craving for sugar. The craving is strong, sometimes almost unbearable. Reassurance that the craving most often disappears after three weeks of careful attention to the diet is enough to help some people through this time. As long as they know that the craving is not something that must be endured forever, they often have enough willpower to stay away from sugar. In a small number of cases, about 200 mgs of vitamin B-2 (riboflavin) is added to the B vitamins already prescribed, and this helps cut down on the craving for sugar or alcohol.

The majority of people who start the diet are able to get through the first stage if they are given enough support and if they are guided as to what to expect. Family and friends may be good sources of encouragement if they, too, understand what to expect.

Second Stage

The onset of the second stage is dramatic. There is a sudden sense of well-being accompanied by energy and a general absence of most of the original complaints. This is but a short respite, however, since the second stage is characterized by rapid swings from a welcome relief and positive feelings to the presence of all of the uncomfortable symptoms that were experienced in the past. Let me emphasize that these swings from high to low are rapid. The second stage may start with a return of energy for a few hours followed quickly by a return to a state in which the original symptoms are present. Very often, changes occur every 12 to 24 hours, but they may be as infrequent as every several days. It is important for the person experiencing these changes to know that these swings are to be expected. I have seen unprepared patients erroneously assume that everything was normal at the first return of energy. Within 24 hours, they could be found in the depths of despair, not only because this is natural in the second stage, but because the symptoms that they had thought were all gone had now returned. They had misinterpreted this as a sign that they would never be well. Beware false interpretations. The proper interpretation at this time is that the swings in mood

and energy are a sign showing that the treatment is progress-
ing as expected.

The danger in this period is in the natural temptation at
the first dramatic sign that the person feels like he used to
feel to make all sorts of plans, such as dates with friends or
relatives who have been long neglected, or plans to do chores
that have been put aside while waiting to feel better. It is a
terrible mistake to make all these plans since feeling well cannot be assured from one day to the next during the second
stage. The only thing one can be sure of is that the mood and
level of energy will change from one day to the next. In making
plans to do long-neglected activities, the chances are high
that when the day arrives the patient will not feel well enough
to execute the plans. This "failure" adds to the feeling that
he will never be well and only reinforces an already strong
feeling of poor self-esteem. The best advice during the second stage is to live one day at a time. Make no plans. If you
feel like doing something one day, do it, but don't plan anything for tomorrow. This advice is very important at this time
since most people with hypoglycemia have been dealing with
long-standing feelings of guilt regarding their relationships
with family and friends. They have been unable to fulfill satisfactorily their roles as parent, spouse, adult, or child. At
the first signs of energy and lack of depression, most people
have a tendency to move too fast to make up for lost time.
They only end up hurting themselves. Their subsequent dis-
appointments make them feel once again unable to fulfill
their roles.

As the second stage progresses, the changes become less
dramatic. The good days are not filled with as much energy
and zest, but the bad days are not as bad either. There is
more constancy from one day to the next, but it is not yet
at an acceptable level. Many times, patients have characterized the end of the second stage by saying, "I am definitely
better than I was before I started this whole thing, but I am
not well enough yet to settle for the way I feel now."

Third Stage

A constancy of feeling from one day to the next and feeling better than pre-diet but not good enough yet characterizes the beginning of the third stage. While the onset and some of the early days of the second stage may be easily described as spectacular, this quality is lacking at the onset of the third stage. In fact, many people remember their super feelings at the beginning of the second stage and come back one month later and say, "I'm not as well as I was last month." After a short discussion reviewing what has taken place during the month, the current feelings and the original complaints, the patient is usually relieved to see the condition in the proper perspective. I find it useful to explain all three stages of the course of treatment at the onset. Then, as each stage is entered, I remind the patient of the discussion. When reminded of the original expectations, the patient is better able to put his current state in proper perspective. For those who feel they are worse at the beginning of the third stage than they were at the beginning of the second stage, they are able to see that this is an accurate evaluation, but they are also able to see that such a condition is to be expected and therefore represents progression, not regression.

The main characteristic of the third stage is the steadiness of improvement. The main difficulty is that the improvement is gradual, not dramatic, and is so natural that there is a tendency to forget that anything was ever wrong. The danger in such an attitude is that when everything progresses so smoothly, it sometimes seems as if nothing is happening. Under such circumstances, there is a temptation to forget the diet If this happens, then the person usually will go through the experience of learning to recognize how bad they feel and will validate the importance of continuing on a good nutritional program.

Sometimes during this third stage, there is some realization that significant improvement has taken place. The usual experience is to recognize that situations that had previously been put off or managed poorly are now dealt with effectively. A change in one's habits and a lack of the need for naps or extra rest might also be noted. Extra duties in activities that were out of the question before might be taken on without a second thought. Some realization of improvement through life experiences usually takes place during the third stage. Many times, patients have come back amazed at their own ability to handle situations that they remember as being so stressful. It is not uncommon to hear reports of people feeling better not because the situation has changed but because their attitude has changed. In addition to changes of attitude, people frequently find that little problems that had previously been ignored and had grown into large problems no longer exist, because the little problems are handled in an efficient manner at the time they should be handled. As events progress, the person usually has an opportunity to compare his experiences in the present with those of the past and is able to see the differences. If, however, these changes do not take place, it is important for the patient's family, friends, and physician to help by pointing out those areas in which improvement has taken place.

After the Third Stage

Following the third stage, which should be equal in length to the first stage, I usually advise that the patient stay on the diet for the equivalent of a fourth stage. The length of time can be estimated fairly early since each stage takes about the same amount of time. The length of the first stage is the easiest to estimate. It is this time that is usually then allowed for a second, third, and fourth stage. The purpose of continuing the same strict diet during the extra stage is to consolidate the gains and to give the patient experience with his new-found health. The next step in treatment is to individualize the diet, to see just how strict it must remain. To determine what does or does not agree with him, the patient makes his own observations about his generally satisfactory functioning.

SUMMARY

Stage 1: There may be an increase in the severity of the symptoms, and there will certainly be no improvement. Craving for sugar disappears after three weeks if the diet is maintained.

Stage 2: Sudden onset of a feeling of well-being. This stage is characterized by rapid, wide swings in the mood and the level of energy, not necessarily on an equal basis.

Stage 3: Gradual onset characterized by the feeling that everything is better than before treatment but not good enough yet. It is during this stage that significant progress is made in a slow, natural manner.

Stage 4: A stage of continued health that is used as a baseline in order to modify the diet.

Chapter Eight

Expanding the Hypoglycemic Diet

Forever is a long, long time, especially when one is expected to stay on a diet. After seeking the high-quality carbohydrate, moderate fat, moderate protein diet, most people ask, although some are afraid to ask, "Is this forever?" At the start of the diet, it is wise to know that it will probably not be necessary to stay on it forever. After the initial four stages, then treatment progresses to a period that can be described as the detective phase.

The detective phase refers to the next several months when, it is hoped, the patient will learn about himself. With guidance and instruction, the detective work is made easier.

When the diet is first given to a patient, very little is personalized, except in cases where patients have special problems such as allergies. Otherwise, the high-quality carbohydrate, moderate fat, moderate protein diet is the rule for all. It should be obvious, taking our individual differences into consideration, that the amount of high-quality carbohydrates will not be the same for everyone. The initial diet is designed to be low in concentrated carbohydrates for most people. A few will need an immediate adjustment to allow them to have more carbohydrates, and a few will need an immediate adjustment to allow them to have less.

These needs are determined during visits to the physician. Of the majority of people who stay on the original diet, some would be able to tolerate larger amounts of concentrated carbohydrates. It is during the detective phase that the diet becomes personalized to meet individual needs.

The teaching technique that I find best is to tell the patient what to do and what to look for. In this way, experiences are underlined, and the learning process may progress more rapidly than without instruction. I do not suggest what the patient will experience. There may be many differences. I only suggest what and when to observe.

The object is to learn about yourself and your diet in order to have as full a diet as possible while staying as well as possible. During this phase, the diet may be visualized as a bull's-eye target. The bull's-eye is the constricted diet that had been adhered to during the previous months. The outer rings represent changes in the variety and quantity of foods and in the frequency of eating. The ring adjacent to the bull's-eye represents natural carbohydrates that have been restricted— fruits and vegetables, with the exception of sugar-laden dried fruits. If the foods in this ring are tested successfully over several weeks, then a move to foods in the next ring may be tried. This ring may contain foods with greater amounts of carbohydrates in them, or a change in the time of eating. For example, must a snack be taken every few hours? There may be a desire to have larger meals on some occasions. The next ring may include all the absolute "no's," such as sugar, other refined carbohydrates, alcohol, and caffeine.

One's individual biochemistry determines how far out on the target one may go without developing some unwanted symptoms. Most individuals progress to the point where they can have any natural fruits, vegetables, and grains without any difficulty. Some are able to give up snacks without problems. Very few are able to start eating sugar again, but this does not present a large problem since their taste and biochemistry have changed and only rarely is sugar desirable.

So far, we have discussed possible additions to the diet. In order to test these additions successfully, the person doing the testing must be aware of (1) what to look for, (2) when to look for it, and (3) when to test or when not to test.

What To Look For

Generally, if the increased foods cause a reaction, it is described as "like having a hangover." There may be a dullness of sensation, a slight headache, and an awareness of feeling less than optimum. The fourth stage allowed extra time to experience what a healthful life is all about. If this sense of well-being is lost during the detective phase, then the expanded diet is probably not working.

Some people are fortunate to have very specific symptoms that return if the expanded diet is too expanded. During the course of treatment, the common experience is to see an improvement in symptoms that had been long-standing and undiagnosed, such as back pains, chest pains, abdominal discomfort, and headaches. The return of such symptoms is a clear sign that the expanded diet is not working.

When To Look For It

Those who have been very conscious about their diet begin to experiment. They generally feel that one bit of a previously forbidden fruit will lead to an immediate punishment. Not so. I cannot explain why, but the reaction most often occurs the following day. Sometimes, the reaction occurs two days later, and it is not unheard of for a reaction to occur three days later. Because of this delayed reaction, those doing the testing must be informed of when to look for the symptoms. Without this knowledge, there will be a delay in correcting the ill feeling. For example, it would be very difficult to connect a tiredness and headache on a Wednesday with something eaten on the previous Sunday. Our reasoning demands a much closer cause and effect relationship unless we are taught from the outset that a delayed reaction is possible. My experience is that many are able to connect a reaction one day later with going off the diet the previous day, but very few are able to understand the cause and effect relationship when the reaction is separated by three days, unless they have been warned when to look for such a reaction.

When To Test

Because a reaction may take three days to occur, new foods are not tested more often than every three to four days in order to give the body adequate time for the reaction to take place, if there is going to be one. Using this schedule, it is usually not difficult to identify a reaction when it does occur. When the reaction time has been established as 24, 48, or 72 hours, the frequency of subsequent testing should be based on the reaction time for that individual. Usually if a person reacts in 24 hours, they will always react in 24 hours, and similarly for a 48- and 72-hour reactor.

There is also a very definite time when you should *not* test any dietary changes—under stress. Under physical or emotional stress, the person with hypoglycemia is more sensitive to concentrated carbohydrates. There is a greater chance that there will be a reaction if concentrated carbohydrates are given during those times. The physical stress may be as minor as a simple infection such as a sore throat or a common cold. Physical stress might also be brought on by a lack of sleep or too much work, even when the person is happy, such as during a happily anticipated visit from a friend.

Emotional stress is not the sort of ordinary everyday stress that most people are subject to, but is stress above and be-yond that. Worries about family, friends, finances, and quar-rels may add enough emotional stress to further sensitize an already sensitive mechanism to concentrated carbohydrates.

Sometimes individuals don't even know when they are un-der additional stress, but there is a foolproof method of recognizing it in controlled hypoglycemic patients. At times of stress, there is a reawakening of the craving for sugar. This is probably because under stress, there is an increase in the amount of adrenaline that is released, which causes an increase in the amount of stored carbohydrates flowing into the system, which in turn sets into motion the sensitive carbohydrate controlling mechanism, thereby reducing the amount of sugar in the blood and causing the craving for sugar. The person going through the detective phase is warned not to do any testing at all if there is a craving for sugar.

The detective phase may take several months, during which most people learn a lot about their own bodies, in-cluding that their initial strict diet can be varied, and that their metabolism is not static. At one time they may be able to tolerate a very lax diet and at other times the slightest variation from a strict diet may result in multiple symptoms. The difference usually depends on how much stress the per-son is feeling. After they have learned to recognize the ef-fect of stress, many people begin to regulate their diet strictly prior to stressful situations, such as extra work, and thus practice the best medicine of all—prevention.

The most dramatic cases of the body's variable ability to handle concentrated carbohydrates are illustrated by several of my patients who have been on cruises. They usually start going off the diet very slowly. While they are on the cruise, where the major stress might be what to wear that day, they quickly learn that as far as their diet goes they are able to go to the last ring of the target and can eat rich desserts and drink alcohol without any problem. If they have not been warned, the natural conclusion probably will be, "I'm cured and can eat or drink anything." On their arrival home, they continue to eat and drink anything, although usually in smaller quantities than on the cruise. The difference is that at home the stresses are usually greater than they were on the cruise. One's daily routine at the office or home is stressful. The return to reality and the usual daily cares and planning are stressful. In such a setting, it takes only about two weeks to develop symptoms that were experienced before the diet. But after being on a strict diet for two to four weeks, health is usually regained.

A valuable lesson has been learned. The body is not static. It is only through experiences that the individual will be able to regulate food and remain healthy.

The most common mistake made during the detective phase is that the patient fails to recognize or accept when an expanding diet is not working. Numerous times I've seen people expand their diet very carefully almost to their previous state of poor health while never accepting that the expanded diet was affecting the way they felt. Just as the treatment resulted in a slow improvement, when the diet is expanded slowly and doesn't work, the decrease in vitality and health occurs slowly as well. The usual excuse that is given for not accepting that the added foods were not agreeable is, "Well, I was so careful, and off the diet so little, that I didn't think I was feeling bad because of what I was eating."

With most people, however, the detective phase is not a wasted one since they are much better observers after, and much more truthful and careful as well. They often become very protective of their new-found health. For some, having experimented and lost their sense of well-being keeps them from trying new foods. They are encouraged to increase grains and to eat any natural fruits and vegetables, to add variation to their diet. With these additions, the diet is healthful and may be followed by any healthy person to maintain that health.

Chapter Nine

Case Histories
That Reveal the Connection
Between Diet, Disease,
and Personality

Before we go on to Part III of this book, I would like to relate a few case histories to illustrate the symptoms of hypoglycemia and the problems of diagnosis.

Let's look at the case of Bob A., a 15-year-old boy whose eating habits were typical of adolescents—he loved "lots" of ice cream. His family had a strong history of sugar intolerance. His paternal grandmother had hypoglycemia. His mother was an alcoholic (usually associated with hypoglycemia), and several family members on his mother's side had diabetes or hypoglycemia. Strange wonder that this teenager also followed the family trend. His chief complaint was that he felt tired, although he was hard put to say how long he had felt that way. His tiredness caused him to be irritable, which led to his subsequent loss of friends, but he was too exhausted to care. His low energy meant he had low motivation and little concentration, which meant he had a hard time in school. He preferred to just sleep. He had some history of occasional tremulousness, but he could not relate this condition to eating. He frequently felt "low." He did not admit to the use of alcohol. Marijuana? Well, occasionally, when he had enough energy to want to be part of the group.

What an outlook for this young man. No motivation, no friends, no happiness, no joy in life.

He was given a glucose tolerance test, which showed a flat curve, indicating that the blood sugar level failed to rise 50 percent above the fasting level within the first hour.

Fasting— 98 mg percent
$\frac{1}{2}$ hour— 68 mg percent
1 hour— 72 mg percent
2 hours— 73 mg percent
3 hours— 95 mg percent
4 hours— 90 mg percent
5 hours— 100 mg percent

He was started on a hypoglycemic diet and a vitamin B Complex b.i.d. (twice a day); ascorbic acid, 1 gram b.i.d.; and vitamin E, 400 units b.i.d. When he was seen again a month later, he had followed his diet with positive results. He was now able to concentrate and was not plagued by that old tired feeling. His hypoglycemic grandmother said he was alert, responsive, and seemed happier. (The grandmother, who also underwent treatment for hypoglycemia, reported that she, too, was feeling better within two weeks after she began her diet.) Bob's adherence to his diet and the properly prescribed vitamins meant his return to normalcy, friendship, and school achievement.

Don B., 34 years of age and single, complained of having problems in functioning mentally and physically. His medical doctor treated him with popular tranquilizers and sleeping pills, but to no avail. He was beset by a heavy, tired feeling and found it extremely difficult to get through the day, even after he'd slept well. He became neurotic about sleep. He was adamant that a good night's sleep and a lot of it were essential, absolutely!

Two years prior to commencing treatment, he had been well on the way to becoming depressed. This resulted in his quitting his job and going back to school. Temporarily, the change made him feel a little better, but the depression, tiredness, and inability to do anything were returning. He had occasional tremors plus an old, nagging back pain that was an undiagnosed torment. The physical discomfort made him avoid people because they annoyed him and made him irritable, and as he tried to control his feelings, he only became more overcome by stress. For him, life was aimless.

There was no history of diabetes in his family so he had no idea of the effects or dangers of eating sugar. Each morning started with three cups of coffee, each with two teaspoons of sugar. Later, he drank tea at work, with more sugar in each cup. Lunch was a hamburger and Coke. Dinner was a piece of meat with a salad, white bread, and milk. He snacked on fruit.

These are the results of his GTT (glucose tolerance test):

> Fasting— 81 mg percent
> 1/2 hour— 105 mg percent
> 1 hour— 100 mg percent
> 2 hours— 97 mg percent
> 2 1/2 hours— 60 mg percent
> 3 hours— 105 mg percent
> 4 hours— 88 mg percent
> 5 hours— 90 mg percent

At 2 1/2 hours, he became extremely tired and developed a headache. He had been instructed that if prominent symptoms developed during any point of the test that he was to request an extra blood sugar level reading, and, fortunately, the 2 1/2-hour reading was made.

His is a flat curve, but it is particularly interesting to note that at $2\frac{1}{2}$ hours there was a drop of 21 mg percent below the fasting level. This is significant. If the $2\frac{1}{2}$-hour reading had not been made, the data would have yielded just a simple, flat curve. Thus we see how quickly a sugar level can drop and how quickly the body can normalize the level. It is apparent that glucose tolerance tests that only measure the fasting and hourly specimens fail to reveal many cases of low blood sugar. It is essential that the first specimen be taken a $\frac{1}{2}$ hour after the person has drunk the glucose, since there is often a rise at this level. If the $\frac{1}{2}$-hour specimen is not done and the hour specimen approximates the fasting level, one never knows if there has been the necessary rise. Ideally, during the glucose tolerance test, technicians should be in constant attendance and should be trained to draw blood at regular times as well as to draw any extra samples if symptoms occur. On a practical level, however, this is not possible in most physicians' offices and routinely most specimens done at fasting, $\frac{1}{2}$ hour, 1, 2, 3, $3\frac{1}{2}$, 4, and 5 hours will reveal a high percentage of the cases of hypoglycemia. In some instances if the patient notes definite symptoms and if there is at least 15 minutes before the next blood sample, it is wise to request an extra sample from the patient. Recognizing symptoms and when they occur during the test are very important in making the diagnosis.

Don was started on the hypoglycemic diet. One month later, he reported that he felt horrible during the first week, and much better the second week, but he was still dissatisfied because he didn't have enough energy. His sleep improved and his depression was lifting. At that point, he left town for a couple of months.

He returned $2\frac{1}{2}$ months later and reported that he felt fabulous. His energy had increased slowly throughout the $2\frac{1}{2}$ months and he was now relieved of his depression and headaches. His enthusiasm and interest had returned and he had stopped taking all the other medications he had been given for nervousness.

Two months later, he graduated from school and was embarking on art studies. He was then not seen for two years. He reported that about one year ago he began to eat an occasional dessert and to drink diet colas. He began to feel bad again. He noticed a gradual decline that he paid little attention to. Tiredness, depression, and poor sleep were once more becoming his lot. He analyzed himself and went back on the strict hypoglycemic diet. Within a month, he started to feel better but was still somewhat fatigued. He started taking a mild tranquilizer, but that only made him feel drugged. After two months on the diet, he still was not well. He was still troubled with weakness, inability to sleep, headaches, and depression. At this time, he added small amounts of fruit to his diet. Within three months, he was feeling much better. He was no longer depressed, his sleep had improved, and he was again doing well in school. Improvement continued gradually, and in four to five months, he was feeling very well again. The problems were gone and he had two new jobs.

Besides illustrating the importance of the glucose tolerance test and the patient's reactions during the test, this case illustrates what happens after a patient is under control and starts to expand his diet without close attention. Soon, he is out of control and back in the same miserable, unhappy state again. This happens frequently. The patient regresses from a state of good health and rationalizes to himself that it could not be the diet. Until the patient goes back on a stricter diet, general deterioration will continue. But once the diet is adhered to, good health can be achieved and maintained.

Alice Z. was 33 years old and divorced. She complained that people had been making fun of her for about three weeks. She had been evicted. She had left her children and had gone to a motel to live. She felt that spirits from another world were putting themselves into this world. She felt that she was going to be killed. She had noted this feeling in the past and had determined that it was related to her period, when she "became irrational, bitchy and depressed." Prior to this current psychotic episode, she had gone on a strict reducing diet.

Past history revealed that she tired easily but that she also had times of great energy. She had generalized pain including headaches, backaches, and pains in her arms. There was a history of tremulousness and sometimes hunger pains. Family history disclosed an aunt who was a manic depressive. Alice herself had been diagnosed as a schizophrenic.

A glucose tolerance test gave the following results:

Fasting—	100 mg percent
1/2 hour—	133 mg percent
1 hour—	105 mg percent
2 hours—	91 mg percent
3 hours—	46 mg percent
4 hours—	66 mg percent
5 hours—	105 mg percent

Alice was started on a hypoglycemic diet with large doses of vitamins. By the second month, she noticed that she was having better days, although she still felt low sometimes. She noted that there was a definite improvement especially around her period. She stated that she was better able to face her problems and that her ability to concentrate had improved.

Nearly a year passed before Alice was seen again. She had generally stayed on her diet, and became tired and depressed when she didn't. During this time, there were no delusions. She stopped psychotherapy and group therapy.

There was no contact for another year. Then, she reported that when she went off the diet and stopped taking the vitamins, she became tired and had feelings of paranoia. These symptoms stopped bothering her when she got enough sleep. Generally, she is now able to take care of herself and is functioning well in the business world and in her personal life.

Betty B., 34 years old, was told by a physician that she had hypoglycemia. Her symptoms included dizziness, faintness, fatigue, depression, anxiety, and irritability. She had a history of arthritis at 18, but claimed she had no arthritic problems at the present. Her mother was a borderline diabetic.

Betty's glucose tolerance test showed the following:

> Fasting— 86 mg percent
> $\frac{1}{2}$ hour— 133 mg percent
> 1 hour — 99 mg percent
> 2 hours— 91 mg percent
> 3 hours— 85 mg percent
> 4 hours— 47 mg percent
> 5 hours— 74 mg percent

The diagnosis was reactive hypoglycemia (4th hour, 47 mg percent). Reactive hypoglycemia is a term used to describe a blood sugar level that falls below 50 mg percent.

She was started on the hypoglycemic diet. When she was seen one month later, she stated, "There are times when I feel like a human being again!" During the second month, she reported that there were times when she liked herself. By the third month, she felt well except when she had to come in contact with her in-laws.

Psychotherapy was advised, but Betty did not feel like seeing a therapist at that time.

Six weeks later, she reported that she had been feeling well until she skipped a meal one day, at which time there was an immediate return of her symptoms.

The following month, she again did well, until she overdid some extra activities. But when she stopped these activities, she felt well again. She found that when she stopped taking her vitamins, the tired feeling returned. During a holiday, she had some candy, and the feeling of irritability returned.

It was only then that she realized and recognized that the elimination of her prior symptoms was directly linked to her dietary program. Stay on it, feel well. Stray from it, "hello, old symptoms."

People who are going through the treatment often are not aware of their improvement because they do not correlate it to the diet and vitamins. It is only when they stop and consider how they previously reacted to situations that they become aware. Improvement is usually so gradual and natural that it takes a long time to recognize the power of the diet.

Bill W. was 56 years old and married when he first saw me. His wife of 18 months complained that for the past six months he was very irritable and unable to control his behavior. His energy level was high in the morning but deteriorated to very low levels later in the day. He was not confused, and had no pain or aches. Before he consulted me, he had had a general physical examination and had been told that everything was normal. There was no history of diabetes in his family.

Bill had been diagnosed as hypoglycemic years before, but he had been unable to stay on his diet because of his depression. He failed to follow through on any treatment plan.

His behavior caused many people to believe he was either on drugs or alcohol, neither of which was true. However, when he did have white bread or beer, he became erratic, and at times violent. Saturdays were especially bad because he always had a muffin and beer on that day, and then went "crazy." When he was not in his office, he slept a lot. He reported also that he could not maintain a relationship because he felt that people were against him.

The results of Bill's glucose tolerance test were as follows:

Fasting— 110 mg percent
$1/2$ hour— 159 mg percent
1 hour— 250 mg percent

2 hours—98 mg percent
3 hours—78 mg percent
4 hours—82 mg percent
5 hours—86 mg percent

This test showed that there was a rapid decline between the first and second hour and relative hypoglycemia by the third.

He was started on a diet and vitamins. One month later, he reported he was feeling better, he was not groggy or sleepy, and his work was better. He was still awakening at 3 A.M., but he would take a glass of milk and go back to sleep.

One day, he missed taking his vitamins and complicated matters by not keeping up with his snacks, which he'd been ordered to take at 1½-hour intervals. The very next day, his original symptoms were back.

Immediately, he got back on the ordered program and started feeling better again. The day-to-day differences were even apparent enough for his wife to notice them.

During the second month, Bill had his problems, although his energy generally improved. He was able to perform better at work, but he remained somewhat irritable in the evenings.

The third month brought what he was seeking. He was no longer irritable, his energy level was constant all day, he was feeling well, and was no longer depressed, and his work had improved.

With his wife's help, he was able to maintain the discipline necessary to restore him to a healthy, functioning life.

Jane P., a 37-year-old housewife, related a typical story of being unable to find help for hypoglycemia because of widespread misunderstanding of the disease.

Jane's problem was intense headaches and nausea which had lasted for the last year and a half. She had had the standard medical examinations—a neurological work-up including a brain scan, and "everything else." She had been subjected to two glucose tolerance tests, as well.

The first test showed the following:

> Fasting— 94 mg percent
> $\frac{1}{2}$ hour— 79 mg percent
> 1 hour— 79 mg percent
> 2 hours— 81 mg percent
> 3 hours— 93 mg percent
> 4 hours— 94 mg percent

It is sad to report that her own doctor wrote in a letter to me that he suspected that "this possibility represented a starvation situation" and so in all his wisdom he had her take a frequent sugar snack between meals and increase her sugar intake for three days before repeating the blood tests. The second test showed the following:

> Fasting— 100 mg percent
> $\frac{1}{2}$ hour—82 mg percent
> 1 hour—75 mg percent
> 2 hours—92 mg percent
> 3 hours—97 mg percent
> 4 hours—90 mg percent

About a month prior to consulting me, Jane found a book on hypoglycemia and put herself on the traditional high-protein, low-carbohydrate diet. Some days were much improved. Therefore, she was ready to follow the regimen that I prescribed for her.

A month later, she reported that she felt well except when she violated the diet by having cookies. Then she became ill with a condition "just like the flu, but it wasn't."

The following month, she continued to feel very well, although there were occasions when she was bothered. Her family noted the improvement. The headaches she had were less severe, and she was no longer nauseous. She "felt like a new person." She reported that in the past she would have a cola drink only to feel better briefly, and then, much worse.

The following month, she continued to feel well except when she pushed herself physically, when she noted a return of some symptoms.

She was able to report four months later that she rarely had headaches or was nauseous. Her mother, who had been skeptical initially about the whole treatment plan, was now her staunchest ally in keeping her on the plan, and was even making special foods for her.

A few months later, Jane reported that she could control her health very simply. When she adhered to the diet, her health was great; when she deviated, she got the headaches. She was able to establish a clear connection between the foods she ate and her health.

Mona K., a 32-year-old married woman, complained that she had low blood sugar. The year before her visit to me, she had become very religious. In turn, she would curse at God. She repeated the same words, forcing more meaningful thoughts out of her brain. She was frightened of things in general. She felt that her eyes were crossing. Sounds were too loud. Concentrating was difficult. She was frequently confused.

She had been to a "good" medical clinic where she had undergone a complete and rigorous physical examination—except for a glucose tolerance test.

During the initial work-up at the clinic, she was diagnosed as "suffering from psychiatric problems." Psychotherapy was advised.

She was seen a year later, when she again complained about her original problems, as well as a lump in her throat. Again she was told that all her tests were normal. She suggested to the physician that she might have hypoglycemia. She was tested, and the test revealed 41 mg percent at the third hour, at a point when she almost fainted.

She was sent to a nutritionist and put on a low-carbohydrate, high-protein diet. This made her feel better, but "not well enough."

Back to her first visit with me. Her diet was reviewed and she was placed on a very strict hypoglycemic diet, with particular attention to the timing of snacks as well as to the importance of high-quality carbohydrate foods such as cooked whole-grain cereal, and instead of large amounts of protein, she was told to eat moderate amounts. She was also put on a vitamin program.

When I saw her a month later, she noted that although she was not well, she felt much improved. Her thinking was more reasonable, and her husband noted that "she had her old spunk back." This was manifested in her talking back to him, as she had done years ago. She also had regained enough courage to speak to him about his drinking, which was a contributing factor to her problems.

She showed even greater improvement after she joined a yoga class. Physical well-being, as well as mental, is returning at a steady pace.

To encourage Mona, her husband went on her diet, and to their delight his drinking problem diminished, too.

Rose N. was a 23-year-old well-known, very talented actress. She came to see me complaining of being very depressed and of having frequent crying spells. Her depression was so severe that she had made several suicide attempts. She had tried street drugs in an attempt to feel better, but they had no good effects.

In this state, it was difficult for her to be around people and she was very irritable. She gained the reputation of being very difficult to work with, which had adverse effects on her career.

The results of her glucose tolerance test are as follows:

Fasting— 87 mg percent
1/2 hour— 236 mg percent
1 hour— 181 mg percent
2 hours— 36 mg percent

3 hours—45 mg percent
4 hours—61 mg percent
5 hours—73 mg percent

She was put on a hypoglycemic diet and told to take certain vitamins.

In two months, she reported that she was not as depressed. She was regaining stability. She was less angry and irritable. Her crying spells had decreased considerably.

The next month, her feelings fluctuated, but she was always able to carry on her responsibilities.

She was not seen for five months. Although she had not been working, she was not as depressed and she was now able to handle the depression differently. She still had some difficulty with her energy level. She reported that her thinking was clearer.

Recognizing that the diet and vitamins were her last chance for continued mental and physical health, Rose maintained the regimen with few exceptions. Tranquility replaced irritability. Soon the studios realized she was well and she found work again.

This gifted actress was fortunate enough to be spared the end of some other great talents—suicide.

Rose, like other patients, can be helped only if the treatment is geared to the whole person. Psychotherapy cannot help the mind until the body has regained its balance, which is often accomplished through a nutritional approach.

Jack Y., the 16-year-old son of a psychologist, said he ate a lot of sweets and complained of feeling mean and nasty most of the time. He had lots of energy but frequently was "down in the dumps and irritable." He had been a hyperactive child and Ritalin had been the "prescribed" answer to that problem. He had stopped that treatment three years prior to our appointment.

He did have infrequent severe headaches and complained of lower back pain and of occasional pains in his side. His general health was good. Although he had a high IQ, his schoolwork was below average.

He was given a five-hour glucose tolerance test, which he took while he was very tired.

Fasting— 100 mg percent
$1/2$ hour— 162 mg percent
1 hour— 105 mg percent
2 hours— 105 mg percent
3 hours— 95 mg percent
4 hours— 80 mg percent
5 hours— 105 mg percent

Note the drop of 57 mg percent between the $1/2$-hour and 1-hour specimens as well as the 20 mg percent drop below the fasting level on the fourth hour. Based on these findings, Jack was started on the diet.

I saw him one month later. He confessed that on the two days that he didn't stay on the diet he felt "cranky and rotten." He started eating a seven-grain cereal every morning and on these days felt much better. As he began to feel better and less irritable, he thought about himself and his relationships with people. He decided that they were less than satisfactory because he "used to mope around waiting for them to call." He surprised himself by doing more work than he had ever done before. With a better physical feeling and consequently a brightened mental outlook, he was now forming friendships and life was looking pretty good.

Needless to say, he cooperates beautifully in maintaining his diet and is now eating half a portion of a freshly cooked grain cereal every morning with the rest of it as a snack before lunch. During the rest of the day, he stays on the moderate protein, moderate fat, and moderate high-quality carbohydrate diet.

Dana C. was a fearful 24-year-old man who was sent to me

by a psychologist who felt that possibly something was wrong physically. Dana's main complaint was phobias: fears of crowds, fears of captivity, fears of being away from home, fear of getting anxiety, fear of tachycardia (rapid pulse), and fear of fear.

These fears had started about one and a half years before I saw Dana, after he had a bad experience with marijuana. The original fear he had for some time was of death. There was no loss of reality. He didn't suffer from hallucinations, nor did he become prey to impulsive actions. He just had the phobias.

He had had a variety of treatments in his search for relief. He had undergone hypnotherapy, psychotherapy, acupuncture, ECT, and behavioral therapy. His general health was good, and there was no history of mental illness in the family. He did not tire easily. He did not have aches or pains, but he did note some depression.

A five-hour glucose tolerance test showed the following:

> Fasting— 84 mg percent
> $\frac{1}{2}$ hour— 112 mg percent
> 1 hour— 54 mg percent
> 2 hours— 114 mg percent
> 3 hours— 54 mg percent
> 4 hours— 80 mg percent
> 5 hours— 80 mg percent

His test results formed a typical sawtooth curve. It is named sawtooth because when it is plotted on a graph there are two distinct peaks, in this case at the half-hour and again at the second hour. Other abnormalities in this curve are the rapid drop of the blood sugar level between the half-hour specimen and the hour specimen, and again between the second-hour specimen and the third-hour specimen. In addition, there is a drop of 30 mg percent from the fasting level, both at the first-hour and third-hour specimens. All of these changes indicate an abnormal glucose tolerance test.

Dana was started on the hypoglycemic diet and for various reasons did not return for two months. When he did return, he had a great and wonderful variety of excuses for not following the diet at all. He returned later to report he was now keeping to the diet and had noted the following: he was sleeping well, had more sex drive, and was no longer constipated, but he had headaches and pain in the right upper back.

Over the next two months, still on the diet, he showed more energy. Although he still had the fears, he was paying less attention to them. In the next month, he still had headaches and noted the presence of tension. The value of the diet was pounded home to him when he slipped and had a piece of chocolate cake. His symptoms began to return the next day.

After six months on the diet, he was feeling much improved. Although he still had some back pain, his fears had diminished considerably, and, as long as he stuck with the dietary program, he felt much better.

During the entire period, he continued going to his psychologist for psychotherapy and noted that significant beneficial changes were taking place here, too. His psychological improvement again illustrates the necessity for a well-functioning mind and body before significant improvement can take place in psychotherapy. Often nutritional therapy is basic and fundamental to good psychotherapy.

Ron W., a 49-year-old business executive, had been hospitalized with acute labrynthritis two years before seeing me. He stated he had "never been the same since, physically or emotionally." There were pains in his scalp and he was sensitive to loud noises such as barking and traffic. He had been admitted to a large medical school health center and had been diagnosed as having neuralgia and residual labrynthritis.

A few weeks prior to seeing me, he suffered from dizziness and had a work-up, after which he was diagnosed as anxious. His past record was one of good health, and he had taken large doses of vitamins for some time. He complained that he was unable to understand why he had been nervous at times over the past two years.

A glucose tolerance test, done prior to his consulting me, disclosed the following:

Fasting— 95 mg percent
$\frac{1}{2}$ hour— 138 mg percent
1 hour— 147 mg percent
2 hours— 110 mg percent
3 hours— 99 mg percent
4 hours— 51 mg percent
5 hours— 63 mg percent

Even though the glucose tolerance test showed a drop of 44 mg percent between the fasting and the fourth hour, accompanied by symptoms, he was told that his test was normal. Obviously he was diagnosed as normal because none of the levels of sugar had fallen below 50 mg percent. The failure to use the proper criteria for interpretation and the failure to listen to the patient and to look only at the test results resulted in several more months of unnecessary suffering.

After the facts were reviewed, he was put on a hypoglycemic diet. A month later, he started to feel better and his head pains were gone. Within the next month, he showed a change in mood and noted he had been depressed before coming to me. It is interesting that many times patients do not reveal their complaints because they are so used to them. They only recognize the complaints after the problem is gone. Within two months after he'd started the diet, he was feeling much improved and noises were not bothering him anymore.

He went on vacation and was able to go off his diet without

any apparent adverse effects, but he noted, when he came back, that he became depressed and suffered a loss of energy. He was seen at two-week intervals and although he adhered to the diet, he remained anxious and nervous. The original physical complaints of headaches and pain with noise did not recur, however.

After six visits, it was obvious that he was anxious only in relationship to his work. When he was questioned and this observation pointed out, he began to discuss problems involving personnel at work, which he had attempted to "live with." When he finally admitted that these situations were bothering him, he took immediate action at work, and the anxiety and depression disappeared quickly. He was kept on the hypoglycemic diet and had weekly psychotherapy sessions. There has been no return of the symptoms.

This case illustrates the importance, in some instances, of combining physical and psychiatric treatment. The physical, or medical, treatment got Ron to the place where his mind was able to function clearly and his body had enough energy so that he could identify his two problems and be willing to do something about them. In this particular case, although the physical symptoms were taken care of, the continuation of the anxiety in special situations, such as going to work, was a tip-off that more was involved than just hypoglycemia. But again, it was necessary to treat his hypoglycemia before anything could be done about his other real-life problems.

PART III

SECRETS OF BECOMING WHOLE, HEALED, AND HAPPY

Chapter Ten

You Are What You Ate—
Now Become What You Eat

The food we eat influences our minds, bodies, and behavior.

In the following section of this book, you will find information on how the newest findings on diet and nutrition can keep you and your family healthy.

You can rebuild your health by eating wisely.

Most illness is the result of improper nourishment. Just how astonishing the deficiency is is being discovered by doctors and biochemists engaged in orthomolecular psychiatry and preventive medicine.

A very big but very important word, *orthomolecular,* is a word all alcoholics and hypoglycemics should become familiar with. "Ortho" means to straighten. Dr. Linus Pauling, who was Professor of Chemistry at Stanford University, and twice winner of the Nobel prize, used "ortho" to coin the term orthomolecular psychiatry, in order to convey the basic idea that many mental illnesses could be corrected by in effect straightening out the concentrations of specific molecules in the brain in order to provide the optimum molecular environment for the mind.

Many hypoglycemics are sent to psychiatrists after their own physicians have listened to all the varied complaints and have found no other reason for the symptoms than that the patient must be a hypochondriac.

Fortunately, they may be "home safe" for the first time in their lives if their psychiatrist happens to be an orthomolecular psychiatrist, because they treat the patient's *biochemistry*. This is a new and great forward stride in psychiatry.

One's individual biochemistry has been overlooked until now. The minimum daily requirement of vitamins, established by government agencies, is not optimum for all individuals. We are all unique. For instance, the hypoglycemic's daily requirement for some vitamins, food supplements, and basic nutrients may be as much as 20 times greater than other people's. In fact, there have been cases in which the requirements of one identical twin were up to 40 times higher than the requirements of the other.

Much suffering has been ended with this "new thought" biochemical approach. Many people with illnesses that could not have been helped by any other methods have benefited dramatically.

Orthomolecular psychiatry (or shall we call it the biochemical approach?) has helped treat alcoholism, drug abuse, autism in children (who respond chiefly to their own inner thoughts and cannot relate to their environment and often appear to be mentally retarded), hyperkinesis and learning disorders in children, psychosis, depression, anxieties, tension, and sometimes even phobias.

For too many years, the functions of the mind—thoughts and feelings—were thought to be determined solely by one's past psychological experiences. Although psychological experiences obviously are important in determining feelings and thoughts, biochemical and nutritional factors are basic to the normal functioning of the nervous system. In the so-called emotional and psychological disorders, there must be an awareness and investigation of the biochemistry as well as the psyche. Many orthomolecular physicians are finding that the changes in an individual treated by the orthomolecular principles obviate the need for further psychiatric intervention. Sometimes, however, change brought about as a result of orthomolecular treatment is the first step toward effective psychotherapy. There can be no effective psychotherapy without a mind that is able to work and a body that has energy.

Alcoholism, schizophrenia, and obesity, fatigue, asthma, depression, anxieties, some headaches, some epilepsy, and many degenerative diseases such as arthritis and arteriosclerosis are biochemical disorders. Some of these problems may be related to hypoglycemia and/or allergies as well.

Freud himself said that psychoanalysis was not suitable in the treatment of schizophrenics and schizoids (schizophrenia-like patients who may not be overt schizophrenics but who may suffer from social isolation, sexual deviance, eccentric and suspicion-ridden reclusiveness, or from incapacitating attacks of pain or unreasoning fear in response to ordinary business or social challenges). Freud felt that the cause would eventually be shown to be biochemical and that consequently the treatment should be biochemical as well as psychotherapeutic. In spite of this, many analysts tried to treat schizophrenia, alcoholism, hypoglycemia, and many other serious biochemical disorders without treating the body as a whole and without using the orthomolecular approach.

Now that it is obvious that physical illnesses as well as mental illnesses can be linked to nutritional disturbances, it is painful to remember the old-fashioned belief that many psychiatrists and medical specialists still follow: the "drug-oriented treatment is the only treatment."

A variety of diseases including mental illness are now directly correlated with dietary factors. Good health can be better assured if you avoid refined sugars, eat good protein, whole natural foods, plus plenty of *natural* vitamins and minerals, get plenty of exercise, and maintain a good mental outlook.

Once well-balanced meals and enough proteins and complex carbohydrates are adhered to, the patient is able to learn that the subconscious has no reasoning power and believes whatever it is told. We all talk to ourselves, whether we realize it or not. Thoughts are recorded as if on a computer, so we must feed our mind happy thoughts, not fears. When we eat correctly we can be in control of our attitudes. I used to end all my lectures with the following powerful sentence: "You tend to move toward that upon which you dwell . . . so dwell well!" Dwelling well is much easier when the brain is correctly nourished.

Although orthomolecular methods were originally developed for the treatment of schizophrenia, they are now being used to treat a wide variety of mental and behavioral disturbances in adults and children. They are even being used to help solve marital difficulties, which, on the surface, seem to be problems of incompatibility but may, in reality, involve hypoglycemia, alcoholism, and/or other nutritionally based disturbances in either or both spouses.

A side advantage to orthomolecular, and vitamin, therapy has been the awareness it has given us of the need for proper nutrition. The use of supplements and good nutrition involved in our work has made us aware of that need. For example, most of us inherit bodies that work. Then, over the next thirty to forty years, we do all we can to tear down and abuse ourselves. People who wouldn't think of putting the wrong amount of oil or the wrong gasoline into their cars put the worst possible garbage into their bodies, a lunch of ice cream and pie and coffee, for example. They treat their cars, which they will have only for a few years, much better than they treat their bodies, which will be with them as long as they live.

To quote from the very informative "Executive Health" report, which is printed monthly in Rancho Santa Fe, California, by Executive Publications:

STAMP OUT FOOD FADDISM

Food faddism is indeed a serious problem. But we have to recognize that the guru of food faddism was not Adelle Davis, but Betty Crocker. The true food faddists are not those who eat raw broccoli, wheat germ, and yogurt, but those who start the day on Breakfast Squares, gulp down bottle after bottle of soda pop, and snack on candy and Twinkies.

Food faddism is promoted from birth. Sugar is a major ingredient in baby food desserts. Then come the artificially flavored and colored breakfast cereals, loaded with sugar, followed by soda pop and hot dogs. Meat marbled with fat and alcoholic beverages dominate the diets of many middle-aged people. And, of course, white bread is standard fare throughout life.

This diet—high in hydrogenated fats, refined sugar, and refined grains—is the prescription for illness: it can contribute to obesity, tooth decay, heart disease, intestinal cancer, and diabetes. And these diseases are, in fact, America's major health problem. So if any diet should be considered faddist, it is the standard one. Our far-out diet—almost 20 percent refined sugar and 45 percent hydrogenated fat—is new to human experience and foreign to all other animal life. . . .

It is incredible that people who eat junk food diets constitute the norm, while individuals whose diets resemble those of our great grandparents are labeled deviants. . . .

The trouble is not only with our lack of education, but with the failure of medicine to recognize the importance of nutrition. If you have been to a doctor and asked about diet or what vitamins to take, you know the response. He usually tells you to get a "one-a-day" or to "eat right," and that's the extent of the advice. That's because the concentration is on treatment rather than prevention. Doctors aren't really too much at fault, because as we have said, medical schools teach very little about nutrition. Twenty years ago, medical schools taught that it was useless to take large amounts of vitamins because all the extra is excreted. We have come a long way since then.

One of the major reasons we are undernourished is found in the quality of the soil in which the farmer plants. The farms are being overworked, and the chemical fertilizers being used today actually "chase out" many of the good minerals we need. If the nutrients aren't in the soil, they can't get into the vegetables and grains, and as a result, they can't get into us. Our preoccupation with the chemistry, rather than the biology of the soil, has produced its own problems.

If we don't educate our farmers about the importance of organic farming, we will be in for a grave health crisis. They must learn that commercial chemical fertilizers do not make soil fertile. They must learn what fertile soil really is. (Fertility is restored to the soil by crop rotation, plowing under and use of *natural* fertilizers.)

By buying organically grown food, you can express your sentiments against pesticides and chemicals. The word "organic" crystallizes the efforts of farmers who go beyond the non-use of chemicals to speak of their respect for ecological values. Most organic farmers are growing food that way out of love for the land, for its purity, and in hope of being able to preserve and build the soil for the use of future generations. By marketing food under the organic label, organic farmers are in a very tangible way speaking to people beyond the bounds of their farm, carrying outward into society the love they feel for the land. And they are also speaking to the large chemical companies that spread chemicals far and wide with hardly a thought about the harm they can cause.

Many of these farmers do not have access to the media, and certainly do not have the promotional power of the chemical companies. But they speak to society through the food they produce, trying to sway people's opinions by creating superior flavor and by offering fresher, purer, and yes, most importantly, better nutritional value.

The Danger of Food Additives

Studies have shown the variety of "psychochemical types" among patients with varied illnesses, and their response to specialized vitamin and mineral combinations, and an association between food additives and the inordinate overactivity, destructiveness, inability to concentrate, and other abnormal behavior in children with the "Hyperkinetic Syndrome." Of the children placed on diets free of food additives, food colorings, and refined foods, as many as 75 percent showed vast improvement.

The following was an evening TV news program in California:

> Hyperkinetic is the term used for excessively overactive children. They are head-bangers, head-rockers, crib-shakers, and as infants and in school, they may have very short attention spans and they can become disciplinary problems. The State Department of Education thinks that they know what may be causing it—food additives—the artificial flavorings and colorings that are in most prepared foods; candies, puddings, dinners, ice cream, especially soft drinks and even in those colorful candy-flavored vitamins for children. Kaiser Hospital's Department of Allergies did a special study of additives in one school district, and State Superintendent Wilson Riles is impressed with the results. So he has given the Kaiser diet, eliminating additives, to local school districts. Some school lunch programs are being adjusted for hyperactive children. There are about 2,000 artificial additives now used in foods, and according to Kaiser's study, they cause adverse reactions in practically every system of the body, and this is affecting one out of every ten children in this country.

As a concerned individual, what can you do? First, educate yourselves. There are people, such as the late Adelle Davis, who have written many books on the subject of nutrition. She certainly helped educate the public about the problem. We also recommend that you read the works of Dr. Roger J. Williams, who is a gifted biochemist. There are also informative magazines, *Prevention* and *Let's Live,* that disseminate a remarkable amount of nutritional information, and a great book, *Feed Your Kids Right* by Lendon Smith, M.D., as well as other books recommended at the back of this book. Everyone should read everything they can find on this subject and form their own conclusions. It may be wise to compare one source of information against another. But each article you read will help give you a general feel for the person's views on nutrition.

What can you do in the meanwhile? First, "kick" the refined-sugar and refined-flour habit, and substitute whole grains, vegetables, and natural fruits in season. This is the *core* of any sensible natural regimen.

Put these words somewhere in your kitchen as a constant reminder:

CHANGING THE QUALITY OF YOUR
CARBOHYDRATES CAN CHANGE THE
QUALITY OF YOUR HEALTH AND LIFE!

No matter what "scientific" name is applied to any diet that includes refined foods, it is dangerous.

Refined sugar is a foodless product. (See Chapter 11 on this.) All of its nutrients are refined out of it, and it serves only to draw vitamins out of our bodies. It disrupts calcium metabolism and is injurious to the nervous system and teeth.

The second thing to avoid is refined flour and everything made with it, and the third thing to avoid with diligence is coffee and tea and anything else that contains caffeine, such as many soft drinks. White flour, so pure in appearance, offers little in the way of nutrition, and combined with sugar turns into one of the most wasted and empty calorie sources in our entire diet. Caffeine is a notorious villain because it releases fatty acid into the blood. Among other problems, which should be discussed at length, is the growing evidence that caffeine contributes substantially to heart trouble. A recent study showed that those who drink five to eight cups of coffee a day have a 25 percent greater risk of having a coronary attack than those who drink no coffee at all. Of course, caffeine is out for hypoglycemics. Remember the double danger of some carbonated soft drinks that contain caffeine plus sugar!

You can't fool Mother Nature, so eat only natural foods. If you don't know what *natural* means, there are a few rules to go by: If it's in a box, don't eat it. Generally speaking, if it's made by God, it's good and if it's made by man, it's harmful. Learn the crucial distinction between natural carbohydrates, such as those in whole grains, vegetables, and fruits, and the unnatural, in refined carbohydrates, such as in sugar, white flour, and polished rice.

Because of our depleted soil and the processing of our foods today, vitamin supplements may be essential. There is nothing wrong with the one-a-day type vitamins, but you may need more than that. After reading about nutrition, you should go to a health-food store to see what is available. This may be extremely confusing since there are thousands of products that may at first all look alike. Consult the more experienced clerks, who are usually happy to suggest good-tasting and nutritional food products and who can show you the proper multi-vitamin preparation to keep your family healthy. That will serve as a beginning, and as you learn more about it, you can add to your health-food store shopping list. It is well worth the extra time, consideration, and planning that goes into nutritional balance of foods and supplements. It will save you money you would spend on doctors or hospitals, and may very well add precious extra years to your lives.

To quote the brilliant Nobel prize winner in medicine, Dr. Albert Szent-Györgby, "All the benefits from vitamins are not known for perhaps ten years after we start taking them and then we do not know why we feel so good."

So the message is *avoid processed foods whenever possible*. Take natural vitamin supplements if needed and do everything possible to eliminate refined sugar and refined grains such as white flour, white rice, and caffeine from your diet. Eat whole grains, fresh fruits, and fresh vegetables, but don't cook the life out of them. Hypoglycemics should not have fruit during the initial stage. They should only have fruit after a meal, never alone on an empty stomach. Snack on nuts and seeds instead.

Protect Your Hypoglycemic Child

Attention Deficit Activity Disorder is the latest terminology for unruly kids. Behavioral problems may indicate that the child's body is crying out for biochemical balance, which can be accomplished with the proper meals and frequent high-quality snacks of nuts, seeds, etc. Some doctors and teachers, ignorant of brain chemistry, in an effort to control behavior at school, assure the parents that the answer is in making certain that the child is given Ritalin regularly. Yes, the trade name Ritalin is used in counseling. Diagnosis is based on behavior, not an explanation of why. Currently, the following is the accepted treatment for children with behavioral problems: Behavior Modification (Corporal Punishment), Counseling, Medication.

Money influences people. At this writing, CIBA, the makers of Ritalin, partially funds a nationwide support group for children with behavioral problems. The parents are not told of this financial arrangement. The long term effects of Ritalin are still not known. It is so overly prescribed that some children sell it at school to friends for $10 a pill since it is considered a cheap "high"! One child died in Roanoke, Virginia, snorting it even though it was not prescribed for him. Parents are assured, "You haven't done anything wrong, we have the answer . . . Ritalin." Parents certainly must be educated to the alternatives to drugs. Instead of zonking the brain with drugs, give your precious child complex carbohydrates (whole grains and vegetables), nothing sweet, meals of protein (fish, meat, fowl, soy), moderate amounts of fats, no caffeine, and lots of constructive words to build the child's self-esteem. Share this information with other parents. Start up your own crusade for a "natural way" support group. A good first step would be to join the National Health Federation, P.O. Box 688, Monrovia, CA 01017. Also see the Recommended Reading list in back of this book.

Almost like a scene out of *Brave New World,* as this updated edition is being written, a frightening story has just been shown on *60 Minutes.* What an abuse of power. What criminal misinformation! It was all about the "wonders" of—you guessed it—Ritalin! My heart breaks for the children whose parents may be brainwashed into giving this quick but dangerous fix. In this one-sided presentation, not one word was mentioned regarding the kinds of foods the children had been eating.

Brain health comes from the farm, not the pharmacy!

Chapter Eleven

Amazing Sugar Discoveries

With almost half our diet consisting of refined carbohydrates (refined sugar, white flour, pastas, polished rice, and refined cereals), it is easy to understand why this generation is developing more and more degenerative diseases. The life force has been removed from most of our food.

The refined sugars and refined carbohydrates act like "anti-vitamins." Sugar consists of 100 percent naked calories without vitamins. To digest refined sugar, the body must "steal" vitamins and minerals from other previously ingested foods, thus depleting the vitamin and mineral content of the body. So refined sugar is actually a "minus" food. Sugar is not only full of empty calories, but it is harmful to your health as well. In the heating and recrystallization of the natural sugar cane, something is altered that causes the refined product to become a dangerous foodstuff!

The difference between eating natural, unrefined carbohydrates and refined sugar can be the difference between life and death, for refined sugar is lethal when ingested by human beings.

When there are natural starches and sugars in food, there are also proteins, fats, vitamins, minerals, and enzymes, which together slow the assimilation and the release of sugar to the blood and other parts of the body. No harm results. This is natural. But refined sugar drains and leaches the entire body of precious vitamins, minerals, and enzymes by putting a heavy demand on the body to digest, detoxify and eliminate it.

Read *Sugar Blues* by William Dufty. In it, you are warned about statements made by the "sugar pushers." Remember, they are probably being *funded* by the Sugar Foundation, food companies, or by others who profit by the sale of sugar. Dufty points out that between 1950 and 1956, according to Open Letter II of the Boston Nutrition Society, January 22, 1957, the Sugar Foundation, the Nutrition Foundation, and a number of food companies contributed almost a quarter of a million dollars to Dr. Frederick Stare, who was the head of Harvard's Department of Nutrition.

These sugar-subsidized nutrition "scientists" give us highly slanted and at times virtually untrue statements to promote the sale of sugar.

Disinterested scientists should be particularly cautious about accepting any form of financial assistance from the sugar authorities. Medical students take note: Is your quick, limited course on nutrition being funded by the sugar industry or processed-food companies?

The Pure Food and Drug Laws are frequently regarded as landmarks in the history of social legislation. The government certainly can have no higher aim than the protection of the health of the people. Perhaps biological decline was well along when it became *necessary* to pass laws to prevent people excessively devoted to money-making *from poisoning one another.*

"When people lost sight of the way to live," wrote Lao Tsu, "came codes of love and honesty."

We hope today's medical students won't be brainwashed, but that they will want to know the truth about nutrition.

Meanwhile, Dufty says that Stare expects that sugar will soon be fortified. "Enriching" devitalized sugar with a few synthetic vitamins will be the ultimate perversion. If Dracula drains your blood with his teeth and gives you a vitamin B-12 shot before he flies out the window, would you say you'd been had or enriched?

Fred Rohe of San Raphael, California, has done some extensive and important research work on refined sugar.

> White sugar is a foodless food. By that, I mean that it is devoid of vitamins, minerals, and enzymes, all factors essential for the digestion, assimilation, and utilization of food. White sugar is 99.96 percent sucrose and should be considered a thief, not a food.
>
> It is touted as an energy food, but such propaganda is misleading, for its 'value' can be measured only in calories and they are nothing more than a number, representing the amount of energy produced when a substance is burned. A wet log has calories. But it won't burn. Sugar won't burn, either, not without vitamins, minerals, and enzymes. *The missing elements must be stolen from the real food in your diet or from stored reserves.*
>
> Analysis of molasses, the by-product of sugar refining, reveals that it contains six B vitamins and eight minerals no longer connected with the sugar. So it is these elements in particular that your system must somehow provide to metabolize sugar.
>
> There is plenty of scientific documentation supporting my nutritional put-down of white sugar. Read such books as *Body, Mind, and Sugar* by Dr. E.M. Abrahamson, *Diet and Disease* by Drs. Cheraskin, Ringsdorf, and Clark, *Nutrition Against Disease* by Dr. Roger J. Williams, and many others written by qualified authors and researchers. . . .
>
> If you are eating conventional supermarket food and would like to escape sugar, reading labels will quickly teach you that it is literally everywhere. Often called by different names, sugar, sugar syrup, glucose, corn syrup, dextrose, sucrose, invert sugar, cane syrup, heavy syrup and natural sweetener. The average American eats over a quarter pound every day—because it appears in bakery products, canned and fro-

zen foods, breakfast cereals, even dried fruit and roasted nuts, not to mention candy and soda pop (four teaspoons or more per bar or bottle). Why must everything taste sweet? Because poor quality foods have poor flavor and *nothing* will taste like *something* if it is at least sweet. Sugar is cheap and so, unaware, we have become a nation of sugar addicts.

Until several years ago, I believed that brown or 'raw' sugar was a nutritional alternative to white or refined. Then I took the trouble to visit several sugar refineries in both Hawaii and California. . . .

What I discovered is that brown sugar is white sugar wearing a mask. There are three kinds of sugar which are not white: light brown, dark brown, and kleenraw. Light brown is 88 percent white sugar, dark brown is 87 percent, and kleenraw is 95 percent.

There is another form of sugar being marketed as 'raw' called turbinado. This sugar is approximately 99.5 percent white sugar, the remaining .5 percent being traces of natural constituents which give it an off-white color. Turbinado is even *more* of a hoax than the other so-called 'raw' sugars.

No organic merchant sells white sugar. Nor does it seem to us to be good judgment to ban white sugar because it is refined to the point of foodlessness, containing neither vitamins nor minerals, a definite human health hazard, then turn around and promote products made from 87 percent or more of the very same white sugar.

Since there are two kinds of sugar—cane and beet—there are two methods of producing brown sugars. Cane manufacturers take partially refined sugar containing 97 percent sucrose and remove all but .04 percent of the remaining 3 percent. This 3 percent is in liquid form and by various blendings and crystallization are formed the various brown sugars and the by-product, molasses.

Beet manufacturers buy molasses from cane companies and *'paint'* their white sugar with the cane molasses, the sugar beet by-products being unpalatable.

Sugar refining is largely a mechanical process done in truly huge machines which boil, spin, filter, and separate. Aside from water, the materials which enter the processing are lime,

phosphoric acid and diatamaceous earth. I don't consider
any of these additives where white sugar is concerned because
one thing is certainly true about white sugar; it is 'pure'. No
chemical residues could possibly remain at the end of the
line, so effective is their purification process and consequently, no nutritive value could possibly remain.

But let's look at that purification process. Over and over
again, in our contemporary food industry, we see the same
folly repeated. Precious nutrients created for the building
and maintenance of health are branded IMPURITIES and
removed for us. If it were only a matter of making things
clean, we would be obliged to say thank you very much.

The fact is, however, that those 'impurities' are perishable
nutrients and their removal makes food handling vastly more
profitable. When you remove the nutrition, you also remove
certain problems like fermentation, spoilage, and infestation.
Food has *life*, therefore, is *delicate;* processing quantities must
be balanced against limited shelf life. Foodless food, with little
or no life, has relatively *unlimited* shelf life—they can process
everything in sight, it'll keep for years. . . . *marvelous for cor-
porate health, but disastrous for your health.*

How do the above generalities apply to sugar? To answer
that, one would have to know what *real* raw sugar is. We
already know what the sugar companies think it is; what I
envision exists only in theory—an almost black syrupy mass
of sticky crystals, condensed from cane juice, boiled to kill
bacteria, filtered to remove debris. Such a product would
require special handling, packaging, and storage. It would
be no more than 60 percent sucrose, the balance being
such "impurities" as vitamins and minerals.

One sugar company, with refineries in Hawaii and California, has repeatedly expressed an interest in producing
just such a sugar and actually has shown me a number of
samples from trial runs. The representatives of this company have been thoroughly hospitable; I don't mean to
make them appear as criminals. In order to work with clear

consciences, they have to believe their products are all right, and that's the way they see them. To excuse them further, it can be pointed out that the business they are in was started long before they were born. But maybe before they go, they'll provide us with the "real thing."

Without knowing the facts, some organic merchants have allowed so-called "raw" sugar, or brown sugar, to have a home in their stores. Probably some products containing it are popular. Our interest is not to take the pleasure out of anyone's life, but to play a part in upgrading the quality of American food. If enough of us stop buying junk, the food manufacturers will listen.

In 1979, Americans consumed 125 pounds of sugar per person; the 1995 estimate is 148 pounds each! One out of every four Americans is eating a half-pound of sugar (usually hidden in processed foods) every day! Why is this happening, you may well ask. To quote from the informative writings of Robert C. Atkins, M.D., "It's the fault of the low-fat fanatics who captured the enfeebled minds of the FDA, the Federal dietary dictators who foisted upon us that infernal pasta pyramid. In their rash rush to simple-minded judgment against the supposed dangers of fat, they neglected to warn us that refined carbohydrates are addictive to most people."

Don't use artificial sweeteners. They are harmful! An apparent connection has been found in patients with metabolic, neurologic complications (sometimes convulsions) and the use of aspartame products. *Warning*, aspartame can be found in: instant breakfasts, breath mints, processed boxed cereals, sugar-free chewing gum, cocoa mixes, coffee beverages, frozen desserts, gelatin desserts, juice beverages, laxatives, multi-vitamins, milk drinks, pharmaceutical supplements, cake mixes, soft drinks, table-top sweeteners, tea beverages, instant teas and coffees, topping mixes, wine coolers, and yogurt.

The US Food and Drug Administration recently has allowed the sale of a natural sweetener called Stevia. If cheating cannot be avoided this is your best alternative. If you can't find it, call 1/800/628-5467. The next choice would be Sucanat, manufactured by NutraCane, Inc., 5 Meadow Brook Parkway, Milford, NH 03055.

Diabetics, who are unable to "burn up" sugar, have been found to have a higher rate of coronary heart disease than normal individuals. Through experiments, it has been discovered that the effect of certain foods on the levels of fat and cholesterol in the blood can vary significantly. Sugar seems to increase blood fats when compared with starch and fats.

We're not through exposing sugar yet. It is indeed almost everywhere—hidden, lurking dangerously—in many foods.

Don't skip over the upcoming section just because you do not put sugar in your coffee or tea. Sugar is hidden in many foods.

The type is large for this list so you will not overlook any item. There is sugar *hidden* in the following:

CANDIES
CHEWING GUM
CAKES
COOKIES
PASTRY
DOUGHNUTS
PIES
ICE CREAM, AND SHAKES MADE WITH IT
JELL-O
PUDDINGS
SHERBET
FROSTINGS
SWEET SAUCES
INSTANT BREAKFASTS (weight-reduction liquid diets)
JAMS

JELLIES
SWEETENED GELATINS
SUGAR-COATED CEREALS, AS WELL AS OTHER
    PROCESSED CEREALS AND MOST COMMERCIAL
    GRANOLAS
TANG
GATORADE
CARBONATED SOFT DRINKS
KOOL-AID
CANNED AND FROZEN VEGETABLES, SOUPS, AND
    FRUITS
STEWED FRUITS
SOUP MIXES
TV DINNERS
PEANUT BUTTER (unless it's the health-food type)
CANNED BABY FOODS
COMMERCIAL YOGURT WITH SUGARED FRUITS
    ADDED
ALCOHOLIC COCKTAILS
KETCHUP
MAYONNAISE
SALAD DRESSINGS
PREPARED SAUCES
CANNED AND FROZEN FRUIT JUICES
BREADS

*READ THE LABELS. YOU'LL LEARN WHETHER THE
FOOD CONTAINS SUGAR. IF SO, JUST PUT IT BACK ON
THE SHELF! AND REMEMBER, DON'T BE MISLED INTO
THINKING BROWN SUGAR IS ACCEPTABLE. IT IS COL
ORED, REFINED SUGAR.*

"For every sweet, there is a sour—a bitter," in this case
the significant interference with physical and mental health.

Chapter Twelve

The Truth About Milk

We are fortunate in California to have the choice of what kind of milk we wish to buy. If you are unlucky enough to live in a state that doesn't allow the sale of raw milk (because pasteurized milk lasts on the grocer's shelf longer), you certainly should demand your right to this choice. Make waves any way you can. Write to senators and the governor of your state and fight for your rights! The production of this desirable food should rest upon practical clinical judgment and not upon the preconceived ideas of those who believe that only sterile dead foods are safe.

Besides raw milk, also use the delicious raw cottage cheese and raw milk cheeses. They are excellent sources of nutrition that are made from unpasteurized milk. During the manufacturing process, the milk is not heated to more than 100 degrees. No coloring or preservatives are added. Did you know that the dark orange color non-raw cheddar cheeses have is not natural but from an additive?

Raw, certified milk is the highest grade, safest, purest milk that skill and care can produce or money can buy! It is produced under rigid standards and is easily digestible, making it the ideal formula milk for babies. Mother's milk, of course, is preferred, but raw milk is the next best option.

Milk in this fresh, natural state has a better taste and contains the properties important to good nutrition that are altered when milk is pasteurized and homogenized. For example:

1. A portion of vitamin C (ascorbic acid) is lost when milk is heated. There is also a reduction in vitamin B-1 (thiamine) and vitamin B-12 (riboflavin).

2. Heating animal protein, as in the pasteurizing process, impairs the value of this protein.

3. Heating milk causes the destruction of 90 percent of the enzymes that help the human body utilize proteins, fats, sugars, starch, phosphorus, and calcium.

4. Pasteurizing milk results in the loss of some calcium, phosphorous, and iodine.

An example of the superiority of raw, certified milk is shown in California's requirements for *pasteurized* milk. The maximum allowable bacteria count is 15,000 per milliliter, whereas raw, certified milk must have a bacteria count of not greater than 10,000 per milliliter and it usually is under this. Therefore, it is easy to see that raw, certified milk is virtually perfect.

Did you know that a calf cannot thrive on pasteurized milk? Some of the elements are so changed that they become dangerous. The chemical structure of the protein is altered and its ingestion has been known to contribute to heart disease.

The fat, once it has become homogenized, also becomes a threat. Homogenization allows xanthine oxidase (XO) to enter the bloodstream through the intestinal wall rather than being excreted from the body. When this enzyme reaches the arteries and the heart, it damages the tissue and raises the cholesterol level. This only happens with homogenized and pasteurized milk, not with raw milk.

Why are people in most states forced to drink only pasteurized milk? Because this heating process that destroys bacteria and nutrients cuts down on the need for strict control of cleanliness. This means that pasteurization yields more profit, the milk has a longer shelf life, and the consumer ends up drinking *dead bacteria*.

Why shouldn't all dairies be required to produce disease-free milk like certified dairies do?

There exist in this country today only four certified dairies: Gates Homestead Farms in New York; Mathis Dairy in Georgia; and Laurelwood Acres in northern California, a goat dairy. The largest, Stueve's Dairy in Los Angeles and San Bernardino counties, distributes its raw milk products now in more than 40 states. We hope you live in one of them.

COMPARISONS	CERTIFIED RAW MILK	PASTEURIZED MILK
Cleanliness	Tested daily at an Independent laboratory for the Certified Milk Commission.	Tested twice a month by the Health Department.
Bacteria count for standard plate count		
Milk	10,000 per milliliter maximum.	50,000 per milliliter maximum before pasteurization and 15,000 maximum after.
Cream	10,000 per milliliter maximum.	25,000 per milliliter maximum.
Anaerobic bacteria test	Once a week.	*None required.*
Streptococci test	Once a month.	*None required.*

COMPARISONS	CERTIFIED RAW MILK	PASTEURIZED MILK
Herd tests in Los Angeles County	Each cow is blood tested for Brucellosis before entering the milk herd and receives a blood test at least once a year. Reactors are removed. All dairy cows in California are vaccinated for Brucellosis between the age of four to six months.	Blood tests are made on a herd only if ring tests on milk are questionable. Reactors are removed.
Ring tests on milk for Brucella	Four times a year.	Four times a year.
T.B. skin test	Every 180 days by a state veterinarian. Reactors are removed.	Tested annually. If reactors are found, additional tests may be required. Reactors are removed.
Sanitary visits	Once a month from the Certified Milk Commission.	*No visit required.*
Employee health examinations	All new employees have a complete physical and monthly exams thereafter.	Examination required at time of employment.
Streptococcus throat culture examination	Monthly	*None required.*
Chest X-ray	Once a year.	*None required.*
Stool specimen	Twice a year.	*None required.*

COMPARISONS	CERTIFIED RAW MILK	PASTEURIZED MILK
Keeping Qualities	Bacteria growth in certified milk increases very slowly, for the friendly acid-forming bacteria (nature's antiseptic) retards the growth of invading organisms, bacteria. *Certified raw milk, produced clean and not exposed to air or human touch, usually keeps for two weeks when under constant refrigeration and later will sour.*	Bacteria growth in pasteurized milk (minimum pasteurization temperature is 161 degrees for 18 seconds) will be geometric (rapid). *After pasteurizing and homogeenizing, milk gradually turns rancid, but will never sour. Rancid milk is not palatable.*
Nutritional Values		
Enzymes	All available.	Less than 10 percent remaining.
Protein	100 percent available, all 22 amino acids, including eight that are essential.	Protein-lysine and tyrosine are altered by heat with serious loss of metabolic availability. This results in making the whole protein complex less available for tissue repair and rebuilding.

COMPARISONS	CERTIFIED RAW MILK	PASTEURIZED MILK
Fats (Research studies indicate that fats are necessary to metabolize protein and calcium. All natural protein-bearing foods contain fats.)	All 18 fatty acids metabolically available, both saturated and unsaturated.	Altered by heat, especially the ten essential unsaturated fats.
Vitamins	All 100 percent available.	Of the fat-soluble vitamins, some are classed as unstable and therefore there is a loss caused by heating above blood temperature. This loss can run as high as two-thirds. Vitamin C loss usually exceeds 50 percent. Losses on water-soluable vitamins that are affected by heat can run from 38 percent to 80 percent.
Carbohydrates	Easily utilized in metabolism. Still associated naturally with elements.	Tests indicate that heat causes some changes, making elements less available metabolically.

COMPARISONS	CERTIFIED RAW MILK	PASTEURIZED MILK
Minerals	All 100 percent metabolically available. Major mineral components are calcium, chlorine, magnesium, phosphorous, potassium, sodium, and sulphur. Vital trace minerals, all 24 or more, 100 percent available.	Calcium is altered by heat, and loss in metabolism may run 50 percent or more, depending on the pasteurization temperature. Losses in metabolic availability in one mineral means losses in other essential minerals, for one mineral usually acts as a synergist for another element. There is a loss of enzymes that serve as leaders in assimilation of minerals.

Chapter Thirteen

The Alcohol Addict

Case histories of alcoholics have been written about, filmed, dramatized, and listened to for so long, but the *answer* to the problem has gone unrecognized. Here now is help for the alcohol addict!

Nothing could be more disturbing to the manufacturers of alcoholic beverages than to have their products referred to as drugs. Drinking is a fine American custom—smart, cool, perfectly acceptable. The staunchest citizens of the land spend prodigious amounts of money stocking their home bars and entertaining themselves and others in cocktail lounges and private clubs. Business contracts are signed over martinis, success is toasted with champagne. Drinking is represented as chic, sophisticated, glamorous. Teenagers can hardly wait until they are 18 or 21, when they can legally carry on the great American drinking tradition. It is a fact, however, that one out of every ten people who take up the drinking habit will eventually find himself addicted to it. The person will assume a dependency on alcohol that is as inexorable and as devastating as any drug habit known to man. Over the past several years, many schools have developed a successful antidrug educational program. But now, many teenagers who wouldn't even touch marijuana or other drugs are rediscovering alcohol. Teenage drinking looms as a serious problem.

Those who do not die from alcohol in a direct way may become one of a dozen or more other statistics. They may contribute to the estimated 10 billion dollars in property damage caused by drinking drivers; they may become one of approximately 30,000 who die each year in alcohol-related traffic deaths; they could easily end up as one of the 25 to 30 percent of the medical-surgical patients admitted to metropolitan hospitals throughout the land. Alcoholism plays a significant role in the number of patients admitted to mental hospitals. This sort of information is available in abundance from numerous organizations, but would require a book of its own to recount. But even if all these statistics were pointed out, it would have little effect on the confirmed alcoholic. He is *hooked* plain and simple.

Inroads have been made in the treatment of alcoholics, and the treatment is the same as for patients of a series of other diseases, including diseases with symptoms of hypoglycemia. There is a good reason for this since it has been discovered that most alcoholics have a hypoglycemic condition. It is possible it developed as a result of faulty diet or because of neglectful habits, or it is highly possible that the hypoglycemic condition set the pattern that led to alcoholism.

For years, it was a popular contention that alcoholism was caused by unfortunate environmental situations during childhood, or that it was "a like father, like son" situation. This theory falls by the wayside, however, when many millions of other individuals with similar backgrounds emerge without the problem. It is typical of the alcoholic personality to blame the condition on outside forces. He could lay it on a domineering parent, a personal tragedy, a failure, or simply on a cruel world out there. But no matter what his rationalization is, it stands to reason that the alcoholic is unique among humans. There is some good reason, beyond the psychological, that makes him an addict. His metabolism does not behave normally when there is alcohol in his system. It is more likely that the condition manifested itself because of his eating habits rather than because he was neglected or because there were midnight fistfights between his parents.

He could be the victim of what many researchers call the "teenage diet," which consists of a high intake of sugar and other junk carbohydrates with minimal amounts of vitamins, minerals, and proteins. Well-meaning parents start early giving the child the taste for sugar. They use sweets as rewards, and the child then craves sweets. The more such foods are eaten, the more such foods are wanted. The heavy drinker assumes the same craving for alcohol. His appetite mechanism is fouled up.

Since alcohol is a carbohydrate, it seems that heavy consumption of it leads to a craving for other carbohydrates. It may mean turning to nothing but fried potatoes when thoughts of food come to mind. In certain cases, such diets have led to beriberi. This is caused by the terrific loss of vitamin B-1 as it is drained by the junk carbohydrates. The number-one thing to know about good nutrition is the difference between the good carbohydrates and the bad carbohydrates. The good ones are the natural ones made by God or nature, and the bad ones are the ones tampered with by man and consequently those that are devitalized. Because they have been stripped of nutrients, the body must try to utilize it by drawing from itself. The "bad" carbohydrates actually use up vitamins and minerals rather than adding nourishment.

In a recent test, rats were limited to the "teenage diet." They were fed a breakfast of doughnuts and coffee; rolls and coffee for coffee breaks at ten and three; hot dogs, soft drinks, pie, and coffee at lunch; spaghetti and meatballs, white bread, salad, cake, and coffee at dinner. The bedtime snack included cookies and candy bars. Out of 100 rats tested, 80 of them chose diluted alcohol as their beverage in preference to plain water. The other 20 stayed with the water until it was sweetened to the equivalent of a mixed drink, then they, too, switched to the whiskey. When half the rats were put on a nutritious diet, they immediately drank from one-tenth to one-fifth less alcohol. The others who were kept on the poor diet continued to consume the same amounts of alcohol. Within 16 weeks, the rats held to the deficient diet were consuming the equivalent of a quart of alcohol a day. They were addicted. It was also discovered that alcohol consumption was cut one-third when their diets were supplemented with vitamins and minerals. The researchers were convinced that there was something in the diet that influenced how much alcohol was consumed. It is their contention that the craving for alcohol comes from a chemical imbalance created by inadequate diet.

There are an estimated four to seven million alcoholics in the United States, and many organizations rank alcoholism among the three top killers—along with heart disease and cancer. But beyond mere statistics, there is no family in the United States that is untouched by the drinking problem. If an immediate member of the family is not affected, you can be sure that at least an uncle, aunt, or cousin is.

It appears also that what was a severe drug problem among teenagers is rapidly developing into an alcohol problem. Hard drug use is finally on the wane, but alcohol consumption is rising drastically. Some researchers go so far as to suggest that a young person's experimentations into most drugs are of a very temporary nature, but the alcohol habit will more likely remain. The years of prohibition did little to control the flow of alcohol, and those who thirsted for it found it abundantly available. The same is true of drugs; those who must have it usually can get it.

Proper nourishment is the first step in helping the alcoholic. The alcoholic's biochemistry must be straightened out through proper diet plus added vitamins. The recommended diet is the hypoglycemia diet.

Alcoholism usually follows a three-phase pattern: (1) heavy drinking, (2) addiction to alcohol, and (3) chronic alcoholism. The drinker may find himself passing through the phases without his realizing it. Some of the symptoms of the phases are as follows:

The *heavy drinker* finds he is devoting more time to drinking; he sneaks extra drinks of larger alcoholic content; drinks to gain relief from tension; requires more alcohol to achieve the desired effect; considers liquor essential to his well-being; needs it as a crutch in social activities; feels guilty about the heavy drinking.

The *addicted drinker* begins to suffer from faulty memory; drinks compulsively; has narrowed interests; has lowered work efficiency; drinks in the morning and during the day; is absent from work regularly; brags and flashes money; lies to family regarding expenditures; is prone to violent outbursts; has a deteriorating marriage; suffers self-pity, becomes increasingly paranoid; rationalizes his drinking habit; has a diminished sex drive; is unjustifiably jealous; hides in liquor; forgets meals; becomes suicidal; shows signs of severe intoxication even when he has consumed little alcohol, because his biochemistry is so upset.

The *chronic alcoholic* begins to show obvious symptoms, both mental and physical; loses his appetite for food; drinks continuously; develops diseases; has a greatly decreased tolerance for alcohol; suffers from delirium tremens; cannot think clearly; turns to the cheapest sources of alcohol; shows symptoms of brain damage.

Individual variations in nutritional needs are very high. Laboratory tests have shown that some rats on a controlled deficiency diet died within a week while others lingered on for as long as five months. The same is true of humans.

There are two energy-yielding chemicals that are commonly consumed and for which self-selection often fails to work advantageously. One is sugar. The other is alcohol. Children who are raised on soft drinks and who are given the choice will choose more of the same in preference to nourishing food. Adults who commonly consume alcoholic beverages regularly and copiously for long periods of time not infrequently reach the point where they lose interest in nourishing food and have, on the contrary, a prevailing interest in consuming alcoholic beverages.

In each case, the appetite-controlling mechanism in the brain has failed. In children, excess sugar consumption leads to general malnutrition. In adults, excess amounts of alcohol without the proper foods not only leads to general malnutrition but to severe brain damage as well.

The nutritional treatment of alcoholics has been substantially successful. Protein foods along with other nutrients have, in some instances, been fed directly into the stomachs of chronic patients. Massive doses of niacin (B-3) have also been prescribed successfully.

The niacin treatment reduces mood swings and insomnia; it lowers alcohol tolerance and the severity of withdrawal discomfort; and also seems to stabilize the alcoholic's behavior so that traditional treatments can be more effective.

Thiamine has also been used successfully. In one instance, an alcoholic of many years had developed severe brain damage. He was given a highly nourishing diet and 500 milligrams daily of vitamin B-1. He was also given dosages of B-2 and B-3. When he appeared for treatment, the patient was unable to coordinate his leg muscles sufficiently to walk. After three weeks of treatment, he left the hospital on his own power.

It has been found that latter-stage alcoholics are so dependent on alcohol and so unaccustomed to proper diet that they will not, or cannot, feed themselves the amounts required. This is the time when vitamins and minerals can be most effective. After being gradually fed with proper nutrients from supplements and *real* food, however, their health gradually improves and they seem to have little difficulty changing their drinking habits.

Everyone has specific nutritional requirements of carbohydrates, fats, proteins, vitamins, and minerals. If any one of the elements is taken without the others, an imbalanced fuel intake develops. Alcohol, if taken to excess, satisfies immediate energy requirements but drains the body of its nutrition. As an analogy, an automobile might operate, however sluggishly, on kerosene fuel. It might slog along for miles on improper fuel, but finally it begins to falter and will eventually stop. The valves and pistons have been blocked by residual sludge and grime. It is not dissimilar in the alcoholic's body. The organs tend to dysfunction because of fatty degeneration.

Deficiencies in vitamins and minerals resulting from total dependence on alcohol as fuel can be reversed by administering appropriate amounts of supplemental vitamins along with well-balanced whole foods. The diet should be moderate in protein, moderate in total fat, and moderate in good-quality carbohydrates. These carbohydrates should be unrefined, whole, and natural. In other words, the hypoglycemic diet is the one prescribed for alcoholics, and as with typical hypoglycemics, there should be snacks between meals.

There are scores of individuals who have gone on this diet, at least partially, with tremendous success. In some instances, the dependence on alcohol was completely and lastingly eliminated, something a little short of miraculous. In other cases, the change was less dramatic. In fact, anyone who has seriously attempted to follow a sensible nutritional regimen has received no less than substantial benefit. Because of its success in combatting alcoholism, I would not hesitate to recommend the diet to alcoholics and to those who may have the beginnings of an alcoholic problem.

In just about every experiment that has been attempted, the results have been impressive. A balanced diet accompanied by supplemental natural vitamins simply works. There have been few incidents when there was not substantial improvement, although there is never a guarantee that the alcoholic will not slip back into his old faulty eating habits and then into the quagmire of weakness and despair. Thus, constant attention to the diet is always of number-one importance.

What is most surprising is the plethora of doctors and counselors who ignore the results of the research that proves that the alcoholic has a blood sugar problem. Families of alcoholics can resort to the private or public "drying out" clinics, but rarely are the research findings used in treatment. One could pay $500 and much more a day at places where no thought would be given to nutrition, and where, if one were lucky, maybe vitamin B would be given. If it weren't so tragic, it would almost be funny. Take a tour of almost any facility where alcoholics are "treated." There, you will always see a large coffee urn with synthetic cream and refined sugar ever ready to jolt the patients' blood sugar into a false lift only to have it sink again and again and again.

I would like to mention here that the wonderful Alcoholics Anonymous Organization has had great success in stopping alcoholics from drinking. God bless them and their good work; however, their members still suffer the pangs of alcoholism even though they are sober because the problem of diet has been neglected. Coffee and doughnuts are usually available at their meetings. These brave souls have licked the drinking problem the hard way. A marriage of the traditional A.A. approach with nutritional education would be a more nearly perfect approach in the battle against the bottle.

Charles S. had a severe alcoholic problem. Within a year of the time of this writing, he was treated in a hospital by one of the most prestigious doctors in the Los Angeles area. Charles's sister remembered reading about hypoglycemia and insisted that Charles be given a glucose tolerance test. It registered a quite dramatic 50 percent drop from the second to the third hour. When Charles received no special instructions after the test, he asked why. The doctor shrugged and informed him that such readings were subject to personal opinion, and his opinion was that Charles had nothing to worry about. The doctor put him on a diet that came out during the mid-thirties. It included sugar in "reasonable" amounts, and placed no limit on coffee or tea. This behavior is almost the equivalent to handing the alcoholic a barrel of whiskey and saying, "Go ahead, it can't hurt you."

The problem is that there are so few doctors today who know the first thing about nutrition, and few of them even have the desire to learn. They feel if something wasn't included in their limited training course on nutrition in medical school, it must not be very important. It is equally unfortunate that only 5 percent of our doctors know how to read or interpret the results of the glucose tolerance test when it is given, and some don't know how to treat hypoglycemia when it does show up on the test.

Fortunately, Charles S.'s story turned out happy. He took matters into his own hands after he read up on hypoglycemia and put himself on a good diet of natural health foods—whole grains, whole raw milk, small amounts of whole vegetables and fruits, plus frequent snacks of protein in the form of nuts and seeds. His health has dramatically improved and he has gone into business for himself and has earned more money this year than he has ever earned in his 49 years. With his new-found health, he has been able to change his negative attitudes to positive ones.

When it comes to alcoholism specifically, there is much one can do for oneself. Stay on the hypoglycemic diet that is detailed in this book, and give yourself liberal helpings of yeast-free vitamin B and other natural vitamins. In addition, follow this simple nutritional rule: no more than ten percent of the calories one consumes each day should be in the form of naked or empty calories. If 90 percent of the calories one consumes are in the form of wholesome food, malnutrition will not become a part of one's life and one will never pass through a period in preparation for drinking, the *sin qua non* or prerequisite for becoming an alcoholic.

It stands to reason that this is excellent advice for all of us. If the empty calories (processed food and refined carbohydrates) we eat could be kept down to a maximum of ten percent of our daily caloric intake, I believe the whole world could take on a different hue. It could mean the end of the junk-food generation. It could suggest the beginning of a generation of better, healthier people, and with better people—healthy, strong, happy people—the state of the world itself would have to improve, because, after all, "in a healthy body dwells a healthy mind."

Chapter Fourteen

New Ways to Improve Your Appearance, Health, and Life Expectancy

Poor nutrition causes disease!

The food Americans are eating is so inadequate that we must take food supplements in the form of vitamins to make up for the loss caused by food processing. Our food has been devitalized so that it will last on the shelves. That's good for the large corporations' pocketbooks, but lethal for the consumer. The most damaging form of pollution is in our food.

The answer to our nation's rapidly declining health is to eliminate the over-processing of foods and to restore the soil through intelligent organic farming methods, as well as eliminate the chemical additives and poisons from our daily diet.

In 1940, it was estimated that ten percent of the food we ate was processed, while today more than 50 percent of our food is processed. While processing may be necessary for food shipped great distances, it certainly is at a heavy price to food's nutritional value. "Enriched" foods, for example, have from 12 to 40 nutrients taken out of them and only about three are put back.

Another processing step involves the additives. If you

could see what goes into a quart of some vanilla ice cream, you would be appalled; you couldn't even pronounce the names of the additives. In fact, some ice cream is practically *all* additives.

To quote from the very informative book *Please, Doctor, Do Something,* by Joe D. Nichols, M.D.: "The American people can never enjoy proper nutrition until they learn the fundamental value of natural foods of high quality. Snacks made from white flour, white sugar, glucose, and hydrogenated fats must be eliminated. The Five D's—Delicious, Delectable, Death-Dealing Desserts—made from these dead foods must be abandoned."

America is starving for a good loaf of whole-grain bread. Wheat, barley, oats, rye, brown rice, and millet, if grown in well-nourished soil and with nothing removed in milling, are rich in valuable nutrients and should be added to your daily diet. Mix some of each of these grains in one loaf and you've hit the jackpot!

We in California are very fortunate to have a superb chain of health food stores called Mrs. Gooch's Whole Foods Markets. They carry organically grown products, meat raised without antibiotics and without hormones, and all kinds of whole grains and freshly baked breads. Chemicals and sugar are not allowed onto their shelves. Equally great markets are: Real Foods in San Francisco, and Wild Oats in California as well as in New Mexico and Arizona. Stores in other states are Bread & Circus on the East Coast, Whole Foods in the Southwest, To Your Health in Boca Raton, Florida, Fresh Foods on the East Coast, and Nature's North in the Northwest.

The number-one thing to remember is to eat foods that spoil—but be sure to eat them before they do. Of course, for the best in nutrition, use only foods that are organic and natural.

Produce should be grown with natural fertilizers and without chemical fertilizers or chemical sprays.

We must once more eat real food that has been tree or

vine ripened. Do you know how many vegetables are picked before they have ripened only to be gas treated to make them ripen on command? We must get rid of the dangerous chemicals and poisons in our environment and in our foods.

If we do not get the proper nutrition, then we will have to use higher doses of natural supplements to bring us back to health.

You have read about the megavitamin approach to curing disease. Following is a chart showing the recommended amounts of natural vitamins, although this can vary depending on individual bio-chemistry and the severity of the disease. Remember, there is no such thing as a chemical equivalent to natural supplements.

I like this quote from the courageous Dr. Carlton Fredericks, "The next time you encounter the legend 'R.D.A.' (recommended daily allowance) on a vitamin or food label, mentally equate it with a proposal to make bras and false teeth in one size, for manufacturing economy, which would make about as much sense."

THE RECOMMENDED DAILY ALLOWANCES (R.D.A.)	THE MEGAVITAMIN DAILY ALLOWANCES USED TO TREAT SOME DISEASES (NOT A DAILY SUPPLEMENTAL DOSE FOR THE AVERAGE PERSON)
Vitamin E (Alpha tocopheral)	
(Please note: DL on the label means the vitamin is synthetic, but D Alpha, without the L, means it is natural.)	
25 international units	100 to 1,600 international units
Vitamin C	
55 mg for adult women;	
	4 grams or more
60 mg for adult men	

THE RECOMMENDED DAILY ALLOWANCES (R.D.A.)	THE MEGAVITAMIN DAILY ALLOWANCES USED TO TREAT SOME DISEASES (NOT A DAILY SUPPLEMENTAL DOSE FOR THE AVERAGE PERSON)
Vitamin B-3 (niacin)	
13 mg for adult women;	
	4 grams
17 mg for adult men	
Vitamin B-6 (pyridoxine)	
2mg	200 mg

As you can see, the megavitamin dosages of vitamin B-3 is 307 times the recommended daily allowance. The B-6 dosage is increased by 100 percent.

The following is a letter from Dr. Alan H. Nittler, author of *A New Breed of Doctor,* published by Pyramid House, written to me when I asked his views concerning natural versus synthetic vitamins.

Dear Jeraldine:

It is my considered opinion that synthetic supplements and "foods" are not the same as the natural and organic counterparts. When I use these latter terms, I mean them as we do and not the technical meanings, ergo that anything containing carbon is an organic compound. A food is defined as a substance which contains nutrients along with the associated factors which allow the substance to be metabolized without depletion of bodily reserves in other areas. Synthetic vitamins and supplements do not contain the naturally associated synergistic micronutrients which allow full metabolism to take place independent of other reserves in the body. They cause depletion of vital nutrients in other areas which must be accounted for in the overall metabolism of the organism.

Natural and organic foods are those which are grown without the assistance of synthetic fertilizers, pesticides, preservatives, et al. They do contain the naturally associated synergistic micronutrients that are necessary for metabolism without stealing factors from other body reserves.

Legal vitamin C is ascorbic acid and it does contain power and maybe even the majority power of the vitamin C complex. But it is not the complex because it is a pure chemical. The chemist considers the naturally associated synergistic micronutrients as contaminants while the nutritionist considers them the *basic factors of life itself.*

Hope that this is specific enough for your purposes. If not, let me know since this is a point which must be sustained at all levels of understanding. The brainwashing must stop and we can really challenge it here.

Now, ordinary ascorbic acid as extracted from natural sources or as extracted or manufactured from coal tar derivatives are not different from each other. They are the same chemically. But this is only talking about pure ascorbic acid and not the C complex.

Sincerely yours,
Alan H. Nittler, M.D.

The selfish group of doctors who are trying to get the government to force us to have a prescription for vitamins are quick to cry that you must be careful because "some vitamins may be toxic if consumed in large amounts." Yes, we do need to know that vitamin A and vitamin D are stored in the body and therefore it is possible to overdose on these, but the appropriate caution can be clearly conveyed via the package label, just as in any over-the-counter medicine. Consider the hundreds of thousands of people who have been poisoned or bled to death by overdosing on aspirin and the staggering number of people who die each year from overdoses of tranquilizers and sleeping aids. The fault is not in the product per se. Did you know that a very large percentage of the patients in hospitals are there because of disorders brought on by medication or therapy their doctors are giving them? These iatrogenic diseases are a direct result of our drug-oriented medical treatment. Drugs are certainly needed in some cases for crisis management, but their continued use may mask symptoms rather than cure them.

Because of the side effects of drugs, the law requires that possible side effects be listed in medical journals—but not on the bottle for the patients to read.

The effects are frightening indeed: nausea, vomiting, tremors, lethargy, coma, rapid heartbeat, confusion, skin eruptions, edema (swelling), constipation, increased or decreased sexual urge, blood disease, jaundice, liver disorders, cramps, headaches, dizziness, stomach irritations, blurred vision, and a multitude of others.

But throughout history, fewer than about 150 people who have taken too much vitamin A over long periods of time have experienced slight discomfort that disappeared after they stopped overdosing on the vitamin. So why the loud warnings and big fuss to try to make the public first get a prescription to buy vitamins?

Generally speaking, the more you weigh, the more vitamins you should have. So infants need very little compared to adults. That is why practically all the cases of vitamin A overdose involve infants. The daily recommended minimum for adults is 5,000 units. More research is needed to find out how much vitamin A is destroyed by DDT, nitrates, and nitrites. It is almost impossible to avoid these chemicals since they are in most processed meats and other foods. Vegetables also contain nitrate if a commercial chemical fertilizer was used instead of a natural fertilizer.

The water-soluble B and C vitamins are very safely passed through the urine if an excess is taken. The same is true of the wonderful vitamin E. Massive doses have been taken without any harmful effects whatsoever, and it is so beneficial for people with heart disease, diabetes, and a long list of other ailments.

Vitamin D is toxic if overdoses are taken, because it is not passed in the urine, but stored. But food sources of vitamin D are scarce. Nature planned for us to get this vitamin from the sun through our skin by the interaction with the sunlight on the skin's oils. That is why it is so healthful to find time each day to be outside, not necessarily sunbathing, but walking or working in the sunlight. If you live where you have little sunlight in winter, then you can take a vitamin D pill every week or so to make up for the lack of sunlight. Four hundred units daily is the recommended dosage. Most milk these days is enriched with vitamin D—400 units to a quart. To prevent SAD (seasonal deficit disorder), buy and use full-spectrum light bulbs. We talk of the importance of light in the following pages.

Vitamin C is a dramatic example of how different individual vitamin requirements can be.

A normal person will spill excesses of this vitamin into the urine when it is taken in large amounts, such as two or three grams a day. Almost 100 percent of all healthy persons will excrete some vitamin C into their urine if they are given four grams. But some individuals who have a great need for this vitamin will not show any traces in the urine even with this high dosage, which is almost 75 times the standard recommended dosage. The individual need for vitamin C has been shown to vary tremendously depending on stress.

Some people (including hypoglycemics) take, retain, and seem to need staggering amounts of vitamin C, B-3, and B-6, and if this need is not met, they become ill. Schizophrenic patients respond especially well to very large amounts of vitamin C.

Children with biochemical imbalances often are hyperactive, autistic, or schizophrenic, but when their individual requirements for natural vitamins, food supplements, and natural foods are met, they respond beautifully and are often capable of enjoying "the good life." Except for a few nutritionally oriented doctors, the most widely used treatment for these conditions is amphetamines, dilantin, dexadrine, and, of course, Ritalin. The sale of Ritalin alone has jumped to over $14 million within the last year. This drug is now causing wall-to-wall havoc in the "Tenderloin" section of San Francisco. Drugs are big business!

The informed doctor seeks the cause of symptoms and believes that their cause is usually a shortage of some *natural* substance. His departure from standard drug treatment was summed up by the brilliant Dr. Roger Williams: "Do you really believe that a headache is caused by a shortage of aspirin in the body?"

Except for stress, nutrition is the only major factor that can be controlled in most diseases. It certainly should be the number-one target in all treatment. The body reacts according to the kind of food—the kind of fuel—it's provided. High-quality fuel naturally promotes better health, while fuelless processed foods do not. It is as simple as that.

Patients, especially hypoglycemics, are in for a shock if they expect to be nutritionally helped while they are in the hospital. The food served there is an example of the worst type. It is as far as you can get from natural and organic. It is steamed, overcooked, and loaded with sugar and carbohydrates tampered with by man. Of course, in many homes the diet is not much better. Is it any wonder we are having a rapid decline in health? In his best-selling book *New Breed of Doctor,* Alan H. Nittler, M.D., an expert in nutritional therapy, says this about our health: "I find hypoglycemia a common condition in my practice. In fact, I assume it to be present until proven otherwise."

Let's face it, we are a nation of "nutritional illiterates," and the only way we can learn about nutritional therapy is to teach ourselves since there is no other source, such as public schools or universities, that are not funded by the powerful sugar industry or processed-food companies. *Nutritional wisdom must be acquired through self-education!*

When we eat properly, we look better, feel better, produce more, and live longer. The *ultimate* in healthful *productive* long lives is found in the people of Hunza. It is very clear that it is their natural way of eating and living that allows them to stay youthful and active for way over 100 years.

The Hunzakuts eat most of their food raw. They seldom cook their vegetables or fruit. Their fruit comes straight from their gardens and their vegetables directly from their fields—without chemical fertilizers, sprays, or preservatives.

In this "Shangri-la," it is unheard of and unthinkable to spray with pesticides. It is their custom to use only natural fertilizers, which eliminate the need for sprays. Soil that has been nourished naturally stays fertile and doesn't require sprays. It is only when farmers continue to take from the earth without replenishing it naturally that sprays are needed. Poor soil grows poor food, which in turn makes people sick.

The people of Hunza grind their wheat fresh each day to make their nutritious bread called chapatti, made from the natural oil of the ground apricot kernel. The unsaturated fatty acids found in natural oils are important for good health.

There are many kinds of unsaturated oils we can use, but most are now only sold in the processed form. The only two oils that can be used safely since they are unprocessed are raw butter and olive oil. Be sure that the oil is fresh and not rancid. Keep it from air and light.

The Hunzakuts use lots of unrefined, unprocessed oil and remain slim. They also have clear complexions and beautiful hair. The myth that oil makes us fat is one of our tragedies. It's *processed* oils and *processed* carbohydrates that create unsightly fat. If you don't have raw butter available in your state, use unprocessed olive oil.

So you see, in Hunza, good nutrition is the way of life for everyone. Not so, unfortunately, in other places in the world. Americans have to go out of their way to find food that is of high quality and poison-free. Devitalized, over-processed foods are found in abundance in all our supermarkets. The shelves are filled with refined carbohydrates and hydrogenated fats. Peanut butter should only consist of peanuts—period. The kind sold now is far from nutritious. If you can't find just plain crushed peanuts without the junk additives, at least buy the kind that isn't hydrogenated.

The precious natural minerals and vitamins so necessary for good health have been removed from most of our breads and cereals. The essential fatty acids found in natural oils have been destroyed by the hydrogenation process. Heart attacks and strokes result inevitably from this mad "scientific" process.

Eaten out lately? Gone are the days when a small pitcher of raw whole cream was found on the table. Now, if you are lucky, you may be served pasteurized, devitalized cream, but more likely you will be slipped "the big lie"—the supposedly cholesterol-free "fat-preventing" nondairy creamer. Sometime, take a magnifying glass and read what this non-food consists of. The tiny, tiny print will probably read like this: water, hydrogenated coconut oil, sodium caseinate, sugar, dipotassium phosphate, propylene, glycol monostearate, polysorbate 60, stearayl lactylate, salt, artificial flavor, color, or some other such poisons. Who in his right mind would prefer such junk to delicious and health-giving whole natural cream? No *informed* person would, not as long as he had eyes good enough to read this small print. Read all labels please!

Remember, food in a box is usually overly processed and devitalized and contains only empty calories. Because these overly processed foods are "fake" foods, they are actually the most expensive foods in America today. The consumer is paying for the process to remove the vitamins and minerals so that the foods will last on the grocers' shelves. Save money by buying whole food. It is better to pay a little more for a good loaf of whole-wheat bread without chemicals (think of chemicals as embalming fluid) than to buy a worthless loaf of "enriched" white bread. You will save on doctor, dentist, and drug bills and also be able to enjoy life more.

If you are interested in maintaining your good health, eating out may pose a problem. Restaurants must be chosen carefully. Many large-chain restaurants have only a few items on their menus, and if you look carefully when the food is served, the size of the portions and the appearance of the food will seem to be exactly alike from one plate to another. The advantage for the restaurant is that they can control portions. When the portions look exactly the same, generally the foods have been processed by taking it apart and reconstituting it, for example, as is done to veal chops and certain steaks. Foods such as potato chips, hard-boiled eggs, and vegetables such as potatoes may also be reconstituted. The reconstituting takes out some nutrients. Usually some additives are put into the food to enhance either its flavor or its appearance. For a frightening but educational experience, spend a few hours looking over some restaurant and/or food technology magazines. It will give you an idea of what is served in most restaurants.

Fortunately, this is not true of all restaurants. Many restaurants called health-food restaurants will serve fresh food. Most cities also have some very good restaurants that serve healthful fresh food prepared in a way that preserves the nutrients. If you are aware of what constitutes good well-prepared food, you should be able to discover restaurants that will meet your needs. When in doubt, choose a Chinese restaurant.

The Cholesterol Myth

Man has taken unto himself to process oils and liquid fats. Oils and liquid fats are not natural foods in that processed state. The oils have been squeezed from seeds, nuts, cereals, and grains that are generally of such poor quality that they cannot be sold or used for other purposes. And even many of the cold-pressed oils are affected by heat during the processing. Harmful and noxious substances are removed. Then come the additives: coloring materials, preservatives, flavorings, and other chemicals. These additives make the oil look right, taste right, smell right, and pour right.

With these oils and more chemicals and processing, you get margarine. Butter is far superior to margarine. The best, however, is raw certified butter. Nature made the butter, man made the processed oils. Remember butter is better!

Polyunsaturated fats *may* lower blood cholesterol, but they do not lower triglycerides, which are of more importance. The polyunsaturated fats diminish the buildup of cholesterol by driving it into the walls of the blood vessels, which can cause hardening of the arteries. Small amounts of unprocessed fats are good and necessary for the proper assimilation of proteins and other metabolism. But hydrogenation and other processing creates an artificial fat that is foreign to the body and should not be consumed.

Hydrogenated foods are to be absolutely avoided! You must read the labels on foods to be sure that you are not buying any that are solid shortening, such as margarine, commercial peanut butter, or factory-made foods containing hydrogenated fats. This includes most crackers, some roasted and salted nuts, commercial "buttered" popcorn, which usually has no butter at all, and any foods, fried in deep fat, such as potato chips, French fries, doughnuts.

Hydrogenation destroys vitamin E and the linoleic acid (a necessary fatty acid for lecithin production). This process also increases the need for choline and raises the blood cholesterol. *Contrary to the general belief that margarine lowers the cholesterol level, it does not. It raises it!*

The hydrogenation process was brought to this country many years ago solely for the purpose of manufacturing soap, not food. It contains nickel, which is a destructive, heavy metal that clings to the walls of the arteries and contributes to cardiovascular problems.

Essential unsaturated fatty acids are destroyed in hydrogenation and deep frying, and unnatural transfatty acids are formed.

The oils used by the Hunzakuts and people of certain other cultures are expressed by centuries-old methods and not by the high-speed modern methods. Therefore, the oils they use are cold-pressed and not changed in chemical structure by heat. The results are essential oils.

Although butter is essentially a saturated fat, it is remarkably different from animal fat since it contains short fatty acid chains. These short fatty acids are transported directly to the liver rather than through the lymph system. The supply of vitamin E in butter increases if the cow grazed on good grass on good soil.

The word *cholesterol* has become almost as frightening to the layman as *cancer* or *heart disease*. Lack of knowledge only helps create anxiety about this "unknown," which may in turn encourage a person to eliminate too many of the *natural* oils from his diet, thereby denying himself of an excellent nutritional source.

Give the egg a break. It deserves a more important place in our diets than it's given. People are aware of the cholesterol in the yolk, but what most people don't know is the egg also contains *lecithin,* which breaks down the cholesterol. There is a town in Pennsylvania where Italian-Americans have eaten cholesterol-rich foods for years—*not* margarine or hydrogenated fats, though—and they seem immune to heart attacks. They use butter, olive oil, etc. Only those people who started to use hydrogenated oils started having heart attacks. It would be better if we could avoid man-made oils and *stress* rather than give up the important egg.

The level of cholesterol in our blood is not raised or lowered only by the foods we eat. The liver produces cholesterol. If one is getting too much of it from foods, the liver compensates by reducing its production. Cholesterol is necessary to the brain and nerve tissue, in the production of hormones, particularly the sex glands.

Dr. Roger J. Williams, in his book *Nutrition in a Nutshell,* says that cholesterol is associated with fats in food. But he says avoidance of excessive cholesterol in food is not of prime importance, for cholesterol is produced in our bodies even when we do not consume any.

Plain yogurt—daki, leben, kisselomelek or medzoon—has been eaten for over 3,000 years and may help reduce the levels of cholesterol in the blood. (Be careful not to buy the yogurt with sugar and additives, though.)

A story was released on September 11, 1974, from Nairobi, telling of 24 Kenyan Masai tribesmen who had eaten all the meat and milk they wanted and who proved to have low levels of cholesterol and to be free of heart disease. Meanwhile, Western men who eat food that is rich in cholesterol worry about getting heart disease. It was thought that the Masais' secret was that they get extensive physical exercise, but, by accident, researchers stumbled upon their real secret—yogurt made from raw whole milk.

Dr. George Mann of Vanderbilt University has conducted experiments on Americans and has found that if a person consumes a minimum of $3\frac{1}{2}$ pints of whole-milk yogurt a day, it appears to have a definite effect on the person's cholesterol level. The research is still going on, but Mann believes that the bacteria fermenting the milk may produce a fatty acid that stops the body from producing cholesterol in the liver.

Another food that helps lower cholesterol is the apple. Apples have an abundance of pectin, which accounts for its effects. The Italians have fewer coronaries than Americans, it has been found. Possibly this is because the Italians eat much more fruit and leafy vegetables, which also contain pectin. Then, too, apples are filling and leave less room for the other processed foods that increase the cholesterol level in the blood.

No need to pass up nature's good foods because of the cholesterol scare. Stay away from hydrogenated oils (margarine, etc.) and remember that informed nutritionists feel that eggs are a much-needed, healthful food. We should not be overly concerned just because the American Heart Association has given them bad publicity. The brain needs cholesterol. Cholesterol is only harmful when it has been chemically transformed through heat. Never fry any food.

Why Migraine Headaches?

The subject of headaches, particularly migraines, has been dealt with in many books and medical articles, with respect to such factors as emotional problems, stress, eyestrain, allergy, heredity, and fatigue, all of which are sometimes contributing causes.

However, since we have explored hypoglycemia and have found low blood sugar to be a major cause in any number of other illnesses, we want to point to hypoglycemia and faulty diet as important causes of migraine headaches as well.

Studies have shown that the cranial arteries in people who get migraines are especially reactive. Any one of a number of stimuli can set off the attack. Missing a meal can even trigger one.

Low blood sugar, or hypoglycemia, restricts the flow of blood to the cranial blood vessels. When there is conspicuous dilation of blood vessels in the head, either from fasting or from the excessive intake of refined carbohydrates, that may be enough to set off a headache in susceptible individuals.

Some headaches can be caused by certain foods, such as sugar or fruit; hypersensitivity to outside stimuli; an emotional upset; an estrogen imbalance, hypertension, or depression.

Good nutrition and the ability to relax are important to the headache-prone person. Meditation (call it prayer if you like) is a natural way to calm oneself down. Try to continually keep one object or thought in your mind while you meditate. You can gradually train your mind to calm down its random dance so that it can be a more enjoyable and pleasant servant for you.

Yes, There Is Fungus Among Us

There has been new light shed on the cause of hypoglycemia. The yeast Candida Albicans lives in all of us. When stimulated by antibiotics or birth control pills, it may establish an infection known as "chronic candidiasis." In children, following treatment with antibiotics, it can manifest itself as an ear infection and myriad other symptoms. It should be standard practice to order the patient to follow-up use of antibiotics with lactobacillus acidophilus and yogurt.

The listed manifestations of chronic candidiasis are so similar to hypoglycemia that the connection is apparent. For instance, the candida experts list some of its symptoms as chronic fatigue, bloating, diarrhea, constipation, indigestion, recurrent vaginitis (following antibiotics), acne, hives, and other skin problems, lethargy, intolerances to foods and inhaled chemicals, migraine and sinus headaches, allergies, especially bronchial allergies, decreased libido, and premenstrual tension. Hypoglycemia caused by candida overgrowth can affect either sex at any age, including infancy.

Unfortunately, in adults it is too often misdiagnosed as psychosomatic.

It is the allergic toxic response in the brain that leads to emotional manifestations that are really physical but are, unfortunately, treated as psychiatric in its cause.

Anti-anxiety drugs aggravate the hormonal imbalance, and once the psychiatric approach is followed the search for physical causes cease. To quote C. Orian Truss, M.D., the author of *The Missing Diagnosis* (a very important must read), "Some day it will be possible, by laboratory means, to differentiate between physical and psychological causes of symptoms of abnormal brain function . . . and forestalling their erroneous referral for psychiatric treatment." This book was published by The Missing Diagnosis Inc., Box 26508, Birmingham, AL 35226, in 1985.

The Importance of Using Sea Salt

The sea, of course, is where all salt came from originally. The trick is to find a sea salt that does not contain sodium chloride only. A certain amount of sodium is necessary in our bodies, but it must be in balance with the rest of the seawater minerals. In processing, all the minerals except for sodium get thrown away. This material that gets thrown away is called Glauber's salt, and is used by the medical profession to treat certain conditions.

To be sure that the salt will always be "free flowing," even in humid weather, the crystals are coated with sodium silico aluminate. Before this is done, potassium iodide is added to the salt to "iodize" it to provide the "anti-goiter" factor. Iodine, unfortunately, is very volatile—it oxidizes rapidly when exposed to light—so another additive must be added, dextrose, a refined sugar, to stabilize the iodine in iodized table salt. These additives cause another problem. In combination, potassium iodide and dextrose turn the salt purple, so yet another additive must be used—sodium bicarbonate. It is mixed in to bleach out the color.

Natural salts are *not* free-flowing. The least harmful process to help salt from caking is to add calcium carbonate, so check the label.

Erewhon Millers, 8454 Steller Drive, Culver City, California 90230, produces a natural sea salt that is made without additives, sun-dried, and from clear waters off the coast of France. They also make a delicious sesame salt by adding whole sesame seeds to their sea salt. You can use this on any foods that you usually like salted.

The Importance of Roughage

Studies have shown that obesity, diabetes, coronary heart disease, and certain bowel disorders are less prevalent among Africans, who stress the importance of vegetable fiber in their diet, than among North Americans and Western Europeans, who don't.

Diabetes seems to be much more common among people fed on a diet low in fiber. During World War II, a shortage of food supplies forced the British to use a brown, under-milled flour. The incidence of diabetes decreased sharply, apparently as the result of the change in diet.

A diet low in crude fiber may contribute to coronary heart disease, for recent studies have suggested that fiber may reduce elevated blood lipids associated with the disease.

Furthermore, certain diseases—appendicitis, diverticulitis, and cancer of the colon—appear to be more prevalent among westernized people than among people living on diets containing larger quantities of vegetable fiber.

(Caution: when using the following suggested fiber, bran, be sure to drink extra water and make sure the bran is fresh.)

An AP story from Mexico City reads:

DOCTOR BLAMES COLON
CANCER ON BLAND DIET

Dr. H. Marvin Pollard of University of Michigan said, "It used to be bland for everything, but you can see doctors changing to high roughage. Sick Americans are now eating more lettuce and bran cereal and cutting out refined foods and puddings."

Cancer of the colon and rectum is the second largest cancer killer behind lung cancer.

Pollard said one prominent theory blames the high incidence on the American diet. The theory is that we live on too refined a dietary program of refined sugar and refined flour. We live in an era when our bland diet does not provide enough stimulation to the colon.

Pollard said in an interview at the Fifth World Congress of Gastroenterology here that doctors are changing diet prescriptions "as a result of what information is available on possible causes of colon cancer resulting from epidemiological studies." He said the theory holds that a bland diet does not provide enough stimulation to the colon.

Not having enough roughage in the diet slows down the transit time before elimination, and this may be the answer to some of the causes of obesity. Fiber pushes food through faster.

With fiber-rich food, there is less opportunity for constipation, since the transit time through the intestines is much faster. Also, the stool is quite different chemically and bacteriologically when the food is rich in fiber. There is the possibility that the increased retention of the stool in the colon and its different composition may lead to local irritation of the cells of the colon and possibly produce cancer. The differences in the frequency of these illnesses in the U.S. and rural Africa seem to us to certainly prove the point.

We strongly recommend that you increase the fiber intake in your daily diet. We go into diet later in the book, but for now, bear in mind that you should eat many raw vegetables and fruits and only stone-ground whole-grain breads (with no preservatives, additives, or sugar).

The following story, entitled "For Health Don't Go Against the Grain," by Alex G. Shulman, which appeared a few years ago in the *L.A. Times,* is of such importance that it must be quoted. You are urged to read every word of it. Dr. Denis P. Burkitt has made an enormous contribution here. There should be no question in your mind about what harm refined white flour and refined sugar products do to the body. As a surgeon, Dr. Burkitt certainly knows first-hand.

FOR HEALTH, DON'T GO AGAINST THE GRAIN

As I, a practicing Los Angeles surgeon, sat there in the auditorium of one of our major hospitals, I was partially stunned. I could hardly believe what I was hearing and what was happening.

At the podium was Dr. Denis P. Burkitt, a famous English surgeon, lecturing about some of his new ideas on the cause of certain diseases. If this were simply an audience of ordinary people listening to a doctor on health matters, this scene would not have been unusual. But here were about 200 sophisticated, prominent physicians—not noted for their gullibility—listening quietly and patiently, but still skeptically, to a somewhat enthusiastic, slight Englishman with a low-key sense of humor.

He was talking about his 20 years of surgical experience with East African natives and casually dropping such small medical blockbusters as: no appendicitis, no obesity, no diabetes, no hernias, no colonic polyps. These conditions, commonly seen in the United States, are almost unknown among the rural African native.

The facts alone are amazing enough, but Burkitt's explanation was even more startling. To the modern physician it has generally been accepted that, from the point of nutrition, if one receives sufficient protein, carbohydrates and fats, minerals, vitamins and trace elements, these are all that are needed from one's diet to maintain a good state of health. . . .

The profession has, in fact, paid very little attention to the quality of diet, or more specifically, to the physical structure of foodstuffs.

Burkitt's hypothesis is based on his belief that all these

diseases can be prevented by including in one's daily diet sufficient indigestible grain fiber in the form of bran.

As Burkitt continued to speak to the doctors, the earlier condescendingly tolerant smiles slowly began to fade as the audience recognized that they might be listening to an exciting statement; one that dared to wrap up the causes of all those diseases in one neat package.

But how could all these diseases be related to such a simplistic notion? It was all too pat. It had all been stated before—preached and pronounced since man appeared on earth. Basically, it stated that what we are depends upon what we eat.

Burkitt is no stranger to the scientific world. He was recognized and honored for his earlier contributions to the brilliant discovery of the disease that bears his name, Burkitt's lymphoma, an unusual form of malignancy found primarily in the children of Africa. Such a respected scientist needed to be heard and the physicians were listening.

His hypothesis was based on the startling observation that all the ills mentioned above are virtually absent in the rural black African community because of the way their food is prepared.

When grains are ground coarsely and the outer coating of the grain is included in the resultant flour, it is rich in bran. Bran is made up of a long-chain molecule that does not easily become digested. It is this bran which gives brown bread its color. (But we should beware of much of our brown bread which is simply white bread artificially colored brown.)

The facts cited by Burkitt came from unimpeachable statistics collected in the Congo, Kenya, Uganda, Sudan, and in other underdeveloped areas elsewhere such as the Himalayas and in rural Rumania during World War I.

As an example, he used acute appendicitis, a condition almost totally absent in such regions' poorer communities. But when people from these communities move to more developed areas in their countries, or when they move to Europe, their incidence of appendicitis significantly increases. In time, the other colon diseases like diverticulosis of the colon and polyps of the colon and colon cancer inevitably follow.

In 1920, Dr. A. Rendle Short, a British surgeon, described a high incidence of appendicitis at a college that catered to private students with pastry-eating tendencies. He compared their rate of appendicitis with the boys at an orphanage fed on a coarse diet and among whom appendicitis was a rarity.

The effect of the coarse grain diet is to decrease intestinal transit time, that is, the number of hours between eating a meal and its later elimination. By ingenious studies conducted in remote African villages, Burkitt learned that transit time averages 35 hours for the Bantu native compared with 77-100 hours for the average Englishman.

In elderly people in England, this time may be as long as three weeks. It is this high-residue, rapidly moving bulk that is held responsible for the almost total absence of appendicitis. Burkitt claims that in his experience in East Africa, the only people who get appendicitis are those who speak English.

What is said for appendicitis also holds true for diverticulosis of the colon, hiatus hernia and, according to Burkitt, for obesity, diabetes, and even cancer of the colon, all conditions seen very commonly in Western civilized society.

Another aspect of his theory is that in most instances, where communities have changed from a high to low-residue diet, they have increased their intake of sugar and white flour. What role the latter plays is hard to assess, but it is believed that this refined carbohydrate alters the bacterial nature of the bowel contents.

The rise in incidence at the end of the 19th century of diabetes, obesity, and then arteriosclerosis with coronary artery disease, corresponds to the increased consumption of refined carbohydrate, especially sugar, as well as changing to a low-residue diet.

Thus, the overconsumption of refined carbohydrate is believed responsible for both arteriosclerosis and diabetes and the reduction in fiber content for the increased pressure changes within the bowel which cause colon diseases. The bacterial changes of an excessive intake of refined carbohydrate is believed to play a role in increasing colon polyps, colon cancer, and ulcerative colitis.

Burkitt evidently believes that both factors, *i.e.*, low bulk and increased refined sugar and white flour, combine to create so many of civilization's diseases. The exact role of each he is as yet unable to define, and he admits there may be other factors.

And when the doctors heard it all, Burkitt asked them if they knew of a better explanation for these statistics. Since there is no better answer available, no one tried to refute the theory. The doctors, however, did want to know exactly what to buy and how to eat it.

Specifically, he recommends no sugar, no white flour. He suggests whole meal bread, preferably baked at home. For most city people for whom bread-baking is impractical, Burkitt suggests that 2 or 3 teaspoonfuls of 100 percent bran be added to the usual breakfast meal. Naturally, this amount varies with the individual, depending on his response.

According to Burkitt, this will help keep weight down, protect the colon, prevent hemorrhoids—and in short, virtually eliminate many of our common surgical diseases.

As for the doctors, most of them still held their former prejudices, albeit now a bit tattered . . . but in the meantime, there are many Los Angeles doctors suddenly eating an awful lot of bran.

Although the value of fiber in maintaining bowel health is now in the headlines here in the U.S.A., two eminent British surgeons, I. Taylor, M.D., and H. L. Duthie, M.D., published a study showing that daily supplements of bran flakes are far and away more effective than either a high roughage diet or a bulk laxative in the treatment of diverticular disease—a painful and common ailment caused by small pockets or sacs formed under pressure in the colon.

Sixty percent of the patients who received bran were completely symptom-free, compared to 40 percent of the patients taking the laxative and 20 percent of those eating high-roughage foods (*British Medical Journal*). There seems to be no adequate replacement for substantial amounts of bran, the two surgeons concluded.

Bran quickly becomes rancid. If you possibly can, grind your own grain and make your own bran, then you can have freshly ground cereal and fresh bran.

If you are allergic to wheat bran, try the bran from other grains, such as rice bran.

A Caution On Carbonated Soft Drinks

The soft-drink industry has done tremendous harm to the bodies and minds of people all over the world. It has been proven over and over again.

Anyone who is concerned with health should cut out all soft drinks from his diet. Why? They contain caffeine and sugar. Some parents won't give their children coffee but do not hesitate to allow a very young child to drink a Coke! These soft drinks also contain tartaric acid, phosphoric acid, artificial flavoring, additives, and sugar.

If a Veterans' Administration nutritionist's theory is correct, the incidence of gum and bone-softening diseases will sharply increase in the U.S. during the coming years.

"It all has to do with the drastic changes in the past 15 years in the amounts of calcium to phosphorous consumed by Americans," says Dr. Leo Lutwak of the Sepulveda VA Hospital and professor of medicine at UCLA Medical School.

Dr. Lutwak's research, which he has conducted over the past 15 years, indicates that the proportion of calcium to phosphorous in the diet is crucial if people are to prevent bone-softening diseases such as osteoporosis and gum disease, one of the chief causes of tooth loss.

The doctor pointed out at a symposium sponsored by the University of California and the Dairy Council of California that people have been eating too much phosphorous and too little calcium to maintain the optimum balance of the two minerals. His research shows that inadequate amounts of calcium probably are a major cause of osteoporosis.

In the 1950s, the ratio of phosphorous to calcium in the typical diet was about 3 to 1. Today, it is about 5 to 1. "The ideal," he points out, "would be $1\frac{1}{2}$ to 1." The increase in phosphorous is also partly accounted for by the rise in the popularity of soft drinks, most of which contain phosphoric acid as flavoring and preservative.

An estimated 10 to 12 million Americans over the age of 60—most of them women—have osteoporosis or bone decalcification—a major reason for the high incidence of broken vertebrae and broken hip bones in older persons.

Gum disease may be an early indicator of osteoporosis. If it is, then dentists are in the best position to diagnose the earliest signs of the bone-softening disease and stop its progression by encouraging the patient to increase his calcium intake.

The doctor should alert the soda-pop drinkers—yes, even diet-soda drinkers—of the importance of maintaining a balance of phosphorous to calcium. There isn't any calcium in soft drinks. (The body then leaches the calcium from itself, creating decalcification, eventually leading to osteoporosis.) Our concern is that soda-pop drinkers will end up toothless and crippled.

The next time you are tempted to reach for that carbonated soft drink, remember, drinking those sodas carries with it a real danger of tooth and bone problems. Is it really worth it?

Be Aware!

Our health can be maintained only by natural means, not by drugs that only mask symptoms. Medications have side effects and influence our nutrition, resulting in other deficiencies.

Anyone who is taking medications should be aware that

he must increase the amount of nutrients he is getting to make up for the effects of the particular medications. Your physician should be able to tell you what nutrients you need.

There are drugs that cause the loss of nutrients through excretion. For example, patients given some diuretics lose potassium. Potassium performs many important functions in the body, including regulating and maintaining a normal heartbeat. Patients using diuretics must eat foods high in potassium such as celery, bananas, strawberries, or take a potassium compound daily. Note: Vitamin C is nature's natural diuretic and vitamin B-6 helps in some cases. Potassium is also lost when patients take prednisone, a cortisone derivative.

Antibiotics can create problems, too. Therefore, you may need additional B vitamins.

Antibiotics, which are used to kill harmful bacteria, may also kill "friendly" bacteria. Yogurt (the health food supreme) can help replace these friendly flora.

The benefit of yogurt over ordinary milk or buttermilk is that the friendly, much-needed bacteria in the yogurt can live and multiply in the intestinal tract. Yogurt actually can manufacture or synthesize vitamins of the B complex. Other milks such as sour milk or buttermilk are important, but the bacteria found in them cannot live at body temperature nor can they survive in the hydrochloric acid of the stomach.

There was a scare back in 1970 that yogurt caused cataracts. This has been researched and is explained clearly in Beatrice Trum Hunter's book Yogurt, Kefir, and Other Milk Cultures, a Pivot Original Health Book. In tests, the rats that developed cataracts had been fed entirely on a diet not of healthful whole-milk yogurt, but of the commercial type made of milk, from which the butterfat had been removed and to which skim-milk powder had been added to give an acceptable consistency to an otherwise watery product. The galactose content, which is far lower in yogurt made from whole milk, was thus brought into the known cataractogenlc range. The yogurt-induced cataracts could not be distinguished from those in previous experiments by using galactose alone. Also, the metabolic system of rats is different from that of man in that rats have an enzymatic deficiency that does not allow them to tolerate lactose and galactose. Hunter notes that in India, where de-fatted yogurt forms a large part of the diet, the incidence of cataracts is very high.

Now that the controversy resulting from the experiments done by Johns Hopkins rcsearchers Curt P. Richter and James Duke has subsided, we can see that their merit lies in the fact that a danger needs to be pointed out: modern food processing may produce profound hazardous changes in such nutritious, life-giving foods as whole-milk yogurt and other staple foods used throughout the world.

The modification of milk by homogenization (see the chapter on milk) or the modification of oil by pasteurization and by hydrogenation are a few examples of processing that need to be examined carefully in terms of their profound ill effects on nutrition and health.

Shedding New Light

It may seem to be a digression from nutrition, but I would like at this point to stress the importance of full-spectrum light in achieving the ultimate in good health.

The fad of wearing tinted lenses in prescription eyeglasses and building new buildings using tinted glass is one more dangerous instance of man trying to improve on naturc.

In the very informative book Health and Light, by John Ott, scientist and director of the Environmental Health and Research Institute in Sarasota, Florida, Ott points out the dangers of keeping the natural full spectrum of light from our eyes. I don't mean to suggest you should stare at the sun, but extensive studies on the effects of natural and artificial light on man and other living things prove that plants, animals, and man become diseased when they are denied natural light.

Our glands need natural light, too, acquired through the eyes and skin. Learn of the importance of staying away from tinted light bulbs, tinted eyeglasses, tinted windows, and harmful TV rays by reading Ott's book.

Emory Thurston, Ph.D., Sc.D., in his invaluable book, *Nutrition for Tots to Teens (And All Other Ages),* points out that improper light bulbs and harmful TV rays (from some sets) can contribute to hyperkinesis. Adults can be hyperkinetic, too, although the condition is not normally recognized in them.

Tinted windows and pink or colored light bulbs may be flattering temporarily, but to stay beautiful and healthy, use only full-spectrum light. This is not the "soft white" bulb you may be using, for it is not full spectrum.

Change the lights and stop the fights.

Chapter Fifteen

The Vim and Vigor Diet — To Add Zest to Your Life and Attractiveness to Your Body

This eating program regulates your weight. If you are overweight, you will lose weight and if you are underweight you will achieve the proper weight for your body.

Write this sentence and place it on your refrigerator door: *It isn't how much you eat that influences your weight; it is what you eat!*

For a more beautiful body, more vim and vigor and a longer, happier life, the whole family should follow these suggestions for a perfect diet.

MORNING   Any whole fruit (not juice), such as half a grapefruit, before you dress. After bathing and dressing, eat any cooked, unprocessed whole-grain cereal. Alternate between steel cut oats (not oat flakes), Quinoa (which is highest in protein of all the world's grains), hulled millet, amaranth, and buckwheat (some refer to it as kasha). Add to any of the grains one third cup of oat bran. You may want to prepare the cereal the night before. Heat water in bottom of double boiler. While water is heating add the grain, bran, and water into the top of the double boiler and heat on a separate burner. Watch closely until it comes to a boil. Then place the top onto the bottom and turn off the heat. In the morning it will be cooked and may only need to be heated a little, and the whole family can get a perfect start for the day. Make enough for snacks for later in the day.

	Or you may have, if you prefer, one slice whole grain bread with fertile eggs.
MID-MORN-ING	Small serving of cottage cheese (preferably raw), or $1/3$ cup sunflower or pumpkin seeds, or raw nuts (make a mixture of them all and keep them in your home, car, purse, or office for between-meal snacks), or $1/4$ of an apple sliced, with peanut butter or a vegetable. Or reheat any cereal saved from breakfast.
LUNCH	One serving of either meat, fish, fowl, eggs, or vegetarian soy-meat substitute. One vegetable or green salad with any dressing that does not contain sugar or vinegar. The best dressing is extra virgin olive oil with fresh lemon juice. Nuts and seed mixture, or raw cottage cheese, or $1/2$ apple with a small piece of raw-milk cheese, or whole-milk yogurt without sugar. Small portion of fresh fruit.
BETWEEN LUNCH AND DINNER	Fruit with nuts and seed mixture. Sardines make a great snacking food because they are rich in nucleic acids and good protein.
DINNER	Any soup that is not thickened with flour. One serving of any fish, fowl, meat, or vegetarian soy-meat substitute. Vegetables. One slice of any yeast-free whole-grain or seven-grain bread with raw butter. Small amount of fresh fruit for dessert.
BEFORE BED-TIME	Raw milk or soy milk, or the nuts and seed mixture, whole-milk yogurt, or $1/2$ slice of any yeast-free whole-grain bread with any nut butter, or small bowl of millet or any other cooked whole-grain cereal.

PREPARATION

DIET NOTES	Spinach, rhubarb, asparagus, cauliflower, cabbage, and soybeans should be cooked. Other vegetables should be eaten raw. If cooking, use low heat and leave the vegetables a little crisp. Do not cook them to death. If you use rice, make *sure* it is brown. *Never* eat white, polished rice. A small amount of fruit may be cooked or eaten raw, with or without cream, but do not use sugar. Canned fruits should be packed in water, not syrup. Fruits are best raw. Use sparingly.

Lettuce, nuts, and seeds may be eaten quite freely. Never drink fruit juice. It is too concentrated and jolts the blood sugar.

FOR CONSTIPATION—BRAN FLAKES
OR ALFALFA TABLETS

Add bran flakes as often as possible to any foods. Take it plain with milk or add it to soups, meat loaf, and cereal. Alfalfa tablets are also very healthful and helpful for constipation. (They can be found in your health-food store.) Yogurt, unsweetened, and vegetable salad, especially raw celery, is good to alleviate constipation.

ALLOWABLE
BEVERAGES

First choice: water without fluoride. Mountain Dew water or any other bottled water.

Second choice: any herb tea—peppermint, mint, comfrey, white clover, chamomile, fenugreek, papaya, alfalfa, rose hips, mate, lemon grass, sassafras, and many more. Read the label to make sure there is no caffeine.

Third choice: grain coffees because they contain *no* caffeine. Some brands are Pero, Pionier, Cafix, and Postum.

Fourth choice: decaffeinated coffees. Popular ones are Sanka and Brim. There may be others you prefer.

MILK: raw milk is preferable. Soy milk may be used. Carob may be added, and the drink may be served hot or cold. No sugar is needed because carob has a natural sweet taste. For variety, add cinnamon and/or nutmeg.

DESSERTS

Small amount of fresh fruit, unsweetened gelatin, and desserts sweetened only with fruit.

No white sugar. No brown sugar. No kleenraw sugar. No sugar at all. And for hypoglycemics, no honey!

SWEETENERS

Stevia extract, use sparingly. If you must use other sweeteners Sucanat is the second choice.

GRAINS, SEEDS, AND NUTS

Grains, seeds, and nuts are the most important part of a good diet. They contain the life force—the germ.

Sprouting increases the nutritional value of grains and seeds. It's fun to sprout them at home, and it's easy. Mung beans, alfalfa seeds, and soybeans are just some of the sprouts you will enjoy. They are great on sandwiches and perfect for salads and many other ways. Buckwheat, soybeans, sesame seeds, pumpkin seeds, almonds, and peanuts are all complete proteins that are biologically of the highest quality. Other seeds and grains increase their value if they are combined and eaten together.

Grains, seeds, and nuts are loaded with B vitamins, which are good for most degenerative diseases, especially hypoglycemia.

Grains, seeds, and nuts are the best anti-aging food. They actually rejuvenate the cells and prevent premature aging.

Raw, unroasted nuts are preferred. Peanuts, almonds, hazelnuts, cashews, and walnuts are the best. Make sure all nuts are raw and fresh.

Chia, anise, celery, poppy, pumpkin, sesame, sunflower, and flax seeds may be used freely. (Note: Tahini is sesame butter.)

ABSOLUTELY AVOID THESE LOW-QUALITY CARBOHYDRATE FOODS

Sugar, candy, and any other sweets; cake, pie, pastry, sweet custards, puddings, ice cream, Gatorade, Tang, or any other food that contains *any* form of refined sugar. Don't forget, sugar is disguised as corn syrup, sucrose, glucose, dextrose, etc. Soft drinks (colas, etc.) are a double threat because they contain sugar and caffeine!

ALSO AVOID ANY

Coffee, tea, beverages containing caffeine, such as soft drinks of any kind, including diet drinks. Spaghetti, macaroni, or noodles (unless they are made with spinach, amaranth, quinoa, artichoke, or whole grains, which are found in health-food stores). Avoid anything made with refined flours. Instant breakfasts and liquid diet meals, because they all contain sugar in some form. Packaged cereals (especially sugar-coated), *please*, don't inflict them on your young ones. Serve a hot, whole-grain cereal every morning.

SUMMARY

Think of caffeine, sugar, and refined foods as the enemy. Don't be brainwashed by the powerful sugar and processed food industries. Especially guard your children from those commercials on the Saturday morning children's programs! No one needs refined sugar! Get natural sugar from whole fruits.

Caffeine is a drug! Remember, coffee or cola gives you a false pickup, which then drops an hour or two later, sending you to a lower level than you were at before you took it. It also increases the acid level in your stomach, which makes you crave more food than you need. Caffeine can trigger heart attacks, hypoglycemia (low blood sugar), ulcers, allergics, etc.

Chapter Sixteen

Recipes
That Can Change
the Quality of Health
and Life

The following recipes will allow you to serve meals that look great and taste great. Yet they are no great effort to prepare. These foods will give you high energy and normalize your weight while giving you optimum nutrition. They will work for you. They will work for your husband, children, and relatives. They will work for friends. They are great during pregnancy. They are great all the time.

We will emphasize ways of using foods that already exist in nature, not the "improved" products the food industry would have us believe are necessary.

Don't buy "anonymous" foods—foods packaged and intended for human consumption, yet generally devoid of a complete list of ingredients or otherwise useful information.

We will use nutritionally alive foods in these recipes, not foods that have been made to appear and taste fresh through the use of various unhealthful processes.

With this new "whole food" consciousness, we can enjoy the real foods and avoid the bulk of the junk foods on the market.

Buy Food Wisely

You will find that eating these unprocessed foods need not be expensive. In fact, your food bills should be reduced measurably. You are saving on the expensive packaging and chemicals of non-foods, and spending instead on whole, healthful items.

If you don't have a health-food store in your town and if you shop in the supermarket, then our advice is to buy whole foods that have been minimally processed—foods that do not depend on highly processed ingredients and that are free of artificial flavoring and coloring, chemical additives, or other synthetic additions.

Buying food wisely will help people of all life styles—people who already eat well, and also those who now, through poverty or ignorance, eat poorly.

Information You Will Need for These Recipes

Agar-Agar can be replaced with plain gelatin or sodium alginate (derived from kelp).

Grain coffee is made from natural grains that contain no caffeine. A popular one is Pero from Germany. It comes in an instant form and tastes better than regular coffee. Another delicious grain coffee is Pionier from Switzerland.

You will find the following in your local health-food store:

Bouillon and meat flavorings to make broths.

Pasta in all shapes and forms, made from Jerusalem artichoke, whole-wheat, soya, amaranth, spinach, and quinoa flours.

Oat flour, bran flakes, soy flour, canned soybeans, and other products mentioned in these recipes that may be unfamiliar to you.

(NOTE: Sorbitol and mannitol are used in many products labeled as dietetic. Generally, these are not tolerated well by hypoglycemics and are not for those trying to maintain or lose weight. They should be avoided because they are high in the wrong kind of carbohydrates.)

Dextrose, fructose, glucose, hexitol, lactose, maltose, mannitol, sorbitol, and sucrose are all forms of sugar. Dr. Bronner's Barleymalt Sweetener, Stevia and Sucanat may be used in place of it, but very sparingly.

Couscous is a wheat product imported from the Near East, and we will use this grain in some breads, muffins, cakes, etc.

Use sea salt that is sun-dried and that does not have additives. (See "The Importance of Using Sea Salt," in the previous chapter.) This is not the ordinary salt (sodium chloride) found in the average supermarket.

Preparation
Not Destruction

When *roasting* meat uncovered in the oven, use only a very low temperature, around 170° to 200°.

When roasting with a covered pan (this allows for steaming), use a small amount of water, and roast at 350°, no higher. Roasting at high temperatures destroys many nutrients. It is best to cook longer on a low heat.

When frying, brown meat or fowl with butter or olive oil (you may sprinkle with whole wheat or soy flour first), then place the meat in a covered pan or casserole and allow it to steam on a low temperature.

When broiling, leave the door open if you are using an oven. Don't let the meat sit in fat. Hot coals may be used. Turning the meat must be kept to a minimum.

DO NOT fry in the orthodox manner by immersing the meat partially or completely in oil. This method produces indigestible protein bonds.

DO NOT smoke meat, fish, or fowl—this destroys some of the amino acids that are found in these animal proteins.

DO NOT use pressure cookers. Temperatures are too high, which causes the loss of folic acid and B vitamins in vegetables.

DO NOT use microwave ovens. To quote Stig Robert Erland, Ph.D., "The short radio waves excite some of the water molecules in such a way as to produce hydrogen peroxide, which in turn attacks the unsaturated fat. These altered polyunsaturated fats in meat or vegetables can be changed into free radicals inside the body which in turn can produce cancer."

Vegetables as well as fruits should be grown organically. City dwellers are not in a position to have such greenstuffs readily available, but they can purchase these products at health-food stores and other places. The effort is well worth the result. Commercially grown foods should be washed especially well to eliminate any adhering sprays. Peel should be removed if the fruit or vegetable is not grown organically.

Vegetables and fruits should be eaten whole rather than drunk as juices. You get only part of the fruit's nutritional benefit from the juice. Machines that extract juice from a fruit or vegetable and leave a pulp actually refine the food. In other words, many fat-soluble and water-insoluble nutrients get thrown away. In fact, some machines completely emulsify the entire vegetable. Such blending is also undesirable since oxygen is forced into contact with some of the nutrients and partial oxidation of the food can then occur.

Get used to eating raw vegetables and fruits, particularly leafy greens. However, if you do cook vegetables, use little or no water and low temperatures so that the foods appear a little undercooked and crispy, like the Chinese method.

Vegetables should be cooked in the following ways:

Steaming—Place cut vegetables in a small amount of water in a pan, and cover. Cook at low temperatures. The tighter the lid, the less water is needed.

Sautéing (internal steaming of vegetables.) Melt butter in a frying pan, place cut vegetables into a hot pan (do not wash vegetables after cutting), and stir in order to coat the vegetables with the oil. Cover the pan and turn the vegetables intermittently. Cook at low temperatures until just soft when touched with a fork.

Double boiler—Place water in the bottom of a double boiler and bring to a boil. Place the washed and still wet leafy vegetable into the top portion. Do not use a wire basket or a double boiler with holes in the top pan since this extracts water-soluble nutrients.

Soup—Cook at low temperatures. Cook starchy vegetables (tubers) first. Simmer until vegetables are just soft. Do not overcook. The slow cooking crockpots are especially convenient if you are gone all day. Just turn it on low before you leave and it is ready when you return.

Uncooked Grains—Prepare a breakfast cereal in the evening by coarsely grinding the grain in a hand or electric grain or "coffee" mill. Then add enough water to just cover it. Let the water plus the freshly ground grain mixture stand at room temperature overnight. Use about 3 or 4 tablespoons of unground grain per person.

Cooked Grains—There are several seven-grain cereals available at your health-food store. Whole-grain cereal is prepared in a double boiler. It is best to obtain whole grains and to crack them immediately before cooking. Use about three cups of water for every cup of grain, and cook the ingredients over water for about a half-hour. Bring the water in both parts of the double boiler to the boiling point first, then combine the double boiler and add the cracked grain and stir. Cover the pan. Stir once or twice during cooking.

"Give the Egg a Break"

When it comes to nutrition, eggs are the almost-perfect food. They provide all the important vitamins and minerals except for vitamin C, and one egg contains about six grams of high-quality protein.

If eggs from free-running hens are sold in your market, these are the ones you should buy. They are called fertile eggs and are from chickens who *aren't* cooped up in enormous prison-like coops with over 10,000 other birds all eating a "scientific blend" of feed that is loaded with chemicals.

Free-running chickens will probably be a thing of the past one day, so enjoy fertile eggs while they are still available. Eggs from grain-fed, rather than chemically fed, hens are richer in flavor and are less likely to have chemical residue. The cholesterol in the egg has been taken care of by nature with its balance of lecithin.

CHEESE EGGS

1/8 pound natural, unprocessed cheese
2 fertile eggs
1/4 teaspoon pepper
1/4 teaspoon dry mustard
dash of paprika, garlic salt, cayenne pepper

Grate cheese and separate eggs. Add most of cheese and remaining ingredients to egg yolks. Fold in unbeaten whites. Place mixture in buttered Pyrex dish. Top with remainder of grated cheese, and bake at 350 degrees until brown on top. Serves one.

POACHED EGGS A LA CHEDDAR

2 fertile eggs
raw butter
2 teaspoons unprocessed grated cheddar cheese
dash of sea salt and pepper

Lightly grease nonstick egg poacher with butter. Place eggs in poacher and sprinkle with grated cheese and a dash of sea salt and pepper. Cover pan. Cook over medium heat three to five minutes. Serve on two slices of whole-grain or soy bread. Serves one.

CHEESE CUSTARD

1 cup milk (preferably raw)
4 fertile eggs, slightly beaten
1 cup grated unprocessed sharp cheddar cheese
dash of cayenne pepper or paprika
1/4 teaspoon sea salt

Pour the milk into a pan and heat until scalded. Beat the eggs and gradually add the scalded milk, stirring constantly. Add the rest of the ingredients and mix well. Pour the mixture into well-greased custard dishes or a shallow baking dish. Place in a pan with 1 inch of hot water. Bake at 350 degrees for 30 minutes, or until a knife can be inserted in the center and come out clean. Serves two.

CHEESE SOUFFLE

1 1/2 cups milk
6 fertile eggs
1/4 cup raw butter
1/4 cup soy flour
1 teaspoon sea salt
dash cayenne pepper
1/2 pound unprocessed sharp cheddar cheese

Preheat oven to 300 degrees. In saucepan, heat, but do not boil, milk. Separate eggs, putting whites in large bowl, yolks in smaller one. In double boiler, melt butter, then stir in flour, then heated milk, salt, and cayenne pepper; cook, stirring until smooth and thickened. Thinly slice cheese and add to sauce. Stir until cheese melts completely and sauce is smooth; remove from heat. With fork, beat egg yolks until well blended. Stir in a little of cheese sauce. Slowly stir this mixture back into the rest of cheese sauce. With electric mixer or hand beater, beat egg whites until stiff but not dry. Slowly pour in cheese sauce, folding carefully until egg whites are covered. Pour mixture into ungreased 2-quart casserole to within 1/4 inch of top. (Bake any extra mixture in small ungreased casserole.) To form crown, use teaspoon to make shallow path in soufflé mixture, about 1 inch in from edge of casserole all the way around. Bake, uncovered, 1 1/4 hours. Don't open oven while soufflé is baking! Serve at once. Serves six.

DEVILED EGGS WITH MUSTARD

Cut cold hard-boiled fertile eggs in half and remove yolks. Blend with mayonnaise (see salad and dressing section), salt, pepper, and dried mustard. Spoon mixture back into egg whites. Cut halves into quarters. Serve cold on bed of lettuce.

ART'S CONSTANT-STIR EGGS

1 medium-sized leek
8 medium-sized fresh mushrooms, sliced
4 fertile eggs
2 tablespoons whole milk
1/2 teaspoon oregano leaves
1/4 teaspoon ground thyme
1/4 cup any unprocessed cheese

Cook in any cold-pressed oil, but raw butter would be best. Add butter (or oil) to pan, chop the bottom and top of the leek and add to pan. Add mushrooms. Cover, and allow to cook slowly.
Beat eggs. Add milk, herbs, cheese, and mix by hand. When vegetables are partially cooked, add egg mixture to pan. Stir constantly over low heat until desired consistency is obtained. Final product should resemble scrambled eggs. Serves two.

Introduction to Omelets

For variety limited only by your imagination, try an omelet. The omelet is easy to prepare and can be used to wrap any ingredient. But be sure to use fertile eggs. The omelet does not have to be eaten only at breakfast. Why not be different today and have an omelet for dinner and homemade soup for breakfast?

TANGY OMELET

2 fertile eggs
1 tablespoon raw cream
1/4 teaspoon tabasco sauce
sea salt and pepper to taste
butter (preferably raw)

Beat eggs with cream, tabasco sauce, sea salt, and pepper until frothy. Melt butter in pan and pour in egg mixture. Rotate pan until mixture sets. When it is lightly browned, fold and slide onto platter. Seafood may be added to this omelet if desired. Serves one.

SPINACH OMELET

4 fertile eggs
1/2 package frozen chopped spinach or fresh spinach
dash sea salt and pepper
1 tablespoon raw butter

Beat egg yolks and whites in separate mixing bowls with fork or hand mixer. Add salt and pepper to yolks. Then add cooked spinach to yolks and beat. Fold in beaten whites. Grease skillet with butter. Pour in mixture. When it is brown, turn omelet over with spatula, and heat until omelet appears firm. Serves two.

ZUCCHINI AND CHEESE OMELET

1/2 cup sauteed zucchini
2 fertile eggs
2 tablespoons club soda
dash sea salt and pepper
butter for pan
2 teaspoons unprocessed cheese (optional)

Saute the zucchini in a little butter or use leftover stewed zucchini. Break eggs into bowl, add the club soda, salt, and pepper. Beat well with a wire whisk. Grease pan with butter. Pour in the beaten eggs and cheese, if desired. When the mixture begins to thicken, add the zucchini. Cook over low heat until the egg mixture is firm. Carefully fold over in thirds. Serve hot. Serves one.

OMELET ATHANAS

1 leek
1/4 bell pepper—red or green
4 mushrooms
2 garlic cloves (or garlic powder)
4 tablespoons butter
dash marjoram
dash thyme
4 tablespoons raw, whole milk
4 fertile eggs
1/2 cup grated unprocessed cheddar cheese

Grease frying pan with butter. Chop leek, bell pepper, mushroom, and garlic cloves medium fine and add to pan. Cover and let cook on low heat. Add marjoram, thyme, and milk to eggs. Beat well. Add the cheddar cheese and stir. When vegetables are cooked, pour the egg-cheese mixture over them. Cover and let cook until eggs are done. Serve and enjoy this hearty, healthy omelet. Serves two.

OMELET GRECO

4 fertile eggs
1/4 lemon
dash oregano
1 tablespoon butter
sprig of parsley or watercress

Beat eggs well. Add juice from 1/4 lemon. Beat lightly. Add dash of oregano. To 1 tablespoon of butter of your choice, add egg-lemon-oregano mixture and cover. Cook over low heat until done. When you serve, garnish with parsley or watercress. This is a light, fluffy omelet best suited for warm days. Serves two.

Potatoes

One of the good things about potatoes, besides their vitamin and mineral content, is that they can always be bought in their natural state without "destructive improvement." But *stay away from processed potato products!*

Baked potatoes can be enriched with cheese. Just clean the skin, bake the potato, scoop out the inside, and mash, adding raw butter and unprocessed cheese. Put all of this mixture back into the skin. Broil until the top is slightly brown. Eat the skin, too!

SWEET-POTATO SOUFFLE

3 cups cooked sweet potato
1 cup butternut squash
milk (enough to mash with sweet potato and squash to
   make a mixture the consistency of cake batter)
3 egg whites, stiffly beaten
Thicken above mixture with a little whole-wheat flour.
1 teaspoon grated lemon and orange rind

4 teaspoons lemon juice
pumpkin pie spice to taste
enough oatmeal flakes to make a thin layer for the bottom
  of the baking dish

Soak the oatmeal quickly in cold water to soften, then drain.
Lay oatmeal in thin layer in baking pan and toast in 300-de-
gree oven until dry and slightly browned. Mix and mash the
sweet potato, squash and milk; add seasonings and a little
whole-wheat flour to thicken, fold in egg whites, place mixture
over oatmeal base in pan and bake at 375 degrees for 45
minutes, or until browned on top. Serves from four to six.

Introduction to Breads

Perhaps one of the greatest culinary treats is homemade
bread. The picture of warm, homemade bread fresh from
the oven, its aroma wafting through the house, has always
been synonymous with a happy home.

The food revolution, which changed our eating habits,
claimed homemade bread as its major victim. With the coming of store-bought bread years ago, we were robbed of the
nutrient value found in the whole-grain breads made at
home. Vitamins, minerals, and crude fiber were all processed out of our breads. Later, a few of the vitamins and
minerals were put back into the factory breads, and they
were misleadingly called "enriched."

As more is learned about nutrition, more is added to
processed foods. For example, bran was recently added to
some commercial bakery breads, making them "enriched."
Two assumptions can be inferred from this: (1) that those
who process the grains know what is being removed from
them, and (2) that there is sufficient information about human nutrition needs to make it possible to replace the "im-

portant" nutrients after they have been processed out. It is hard to accept these assumptions as true.

If you are interested in good nutrition and good health, you are well advised to avoid all processed foods, even those that are "enriched," whenever possible.

Many breads that do not destroy vitamins in the grinding process, including unprocessed whole grain and stone ground, are available in health-food stores as well as in some large grocery-chain stores. Almost all of these breads do include some sugar or honey, however. Bread without any concentrated carbohydrates (sugar or honey) is preferable. Such recipes are found in this section. The properly prepared homemade bread tastes better than the commercial whole-grain bread. Besides the improved taste, homemade bread also has some more subtle advantages over store-bought bread.

Most people associate homemade bread with holidays, but why wait when you can start baking now.

Life-giving Breads

GRANDMA'S GLUTEN BREAD

(If you have overgrowth of Candida symptoms, eat only bread made without yeast.)

1 tablespoon dry yeast
1 teaspoon sea salt
1½ cups fruit juice
¼ teaspoon caraway seeds (optional)
½ cup oat flour
3 cups gluten flour
½ teaspoon dill weed (optional)

Dissolve yeast and salt in fruit juice in large bowl, add gluten flour, oat flour and dill weed. Mix well into soft dough. Cover with clean cloth and let rise until almost double its size. It is preferable to leave it overnight. Punch dough down and let rise again for 30 minutes. Shape into loaf and place in 9x5x3-inch loaf pan. Preheat oven and bake at 350 degrees for one hour. Makes one loaf.

GRANDPA'S PROTEIN BREAD

1 tablespoon dry yeast
$1/2$ cup warm water
1 cup milk or buttermilk, warmed
$1^1/2$ teaspoon sea salt
1 teaspoon melted butter (preferably raw)
$1^1/2$ cups gluten flour
$1^1/4$ cups soy flour
1 teaspoon butter, melted (preferably raw)
$1/4$ teaspoon caraway seeds (optional)

Combine the yeast and water. Let it stand five minutes to activate yeast. Add the milk, salt, and $1/4$ teaspoon butter and flour. Mix to a soft dough. Turn onto a lightly floured board and knead 20 times. Place in a warm place and cover. Let dough rise until double its size. Knead again and place in 9x5x3-inch loaf pan. Grease top with remaining butter. Cover and let rise for one hour. Bake in preheated 350-degree oven for one hour. Makes one loaf.

FARM LOAF

1 cup soy flour
1 teaspoon sea salt
2 teaspoons baking powder
$1/4$ teaspoon caraway seeds (optional)
1 teaspoon butter (preferably raw)
$2/3$ cups water
4 fertile eggs, separated

Combine all ingredients except egg whites. Beat egg whites

and fold in last. Bake in a 9x5x3-inch loaf pan for 30 to 40 minutes in preheated 350-degree oven. Makes one loaf.

SOY BREAD

6 extra large fertile eggs
1 cup soy flour
$1/2$ cup milk
$1/4$ teaspoon sea salt
$1/3$ cup non-fat dry milk

Preheat the oven to 375 degrees. Beat the eggs well with an electric mixer or blender. Add the rest of the ingredients and stir to mix. Grease a small loaf or bread pan and sprinkle lightly with soy flour; shake out the excess flour. Pour the batter into the pan. Bake at 375 degrees for 10 minutes; lower heat to 350 degrees, and bake for 40 to 50 minutes longer, or until set. Allow to cool before cutting. Makes one loaf.

OATMEAL BREAD

2 cups old-fashioned-style oat cereal
1 cup hot water (but not boiling)
$1/4$ cup oil
$1/4$ teaspoon sea salt
$2/3$ cup non-fat dry milk
4 fertile eggs
$1/2$ teaspoon baking soda
1 cup soy flour

Combine the oat cereal and the hot water in a large bowl. Mix well until the oatmeal is softened. Add the remaining ingredients and stir until well mixed. Grease a loaf pan, then sift in a little soy flour, shaking out the excess after the bottom and sides are lightly coated. Pour in the batter. Place in a preheated 375-degree oven for 15 minutes, then bake at 325 degrees for 45 minutes. Makes one loaf.

ALL PURPOSE EGG BREAD

6 fertile eggs
1 cup oat flour
1 teaspoon sea salt
1 cup soy flour
½ cup non-fat dry milk
1 teaspoon baking powder
1 cup water
1 cup wheat germ
sesame seeds as needed

Beat the eggs and set aside. In a large bowl, sift together the dry ingredients except for the wheat germ and sesame seeds. Gradually beat in the eggs, then the water. Last, mix in the wheat germ, mixing well. Grease a large loaf pan, then dust lightly with soy flour, shaking out the excess. Pour batter into the pan, and sprinkle the top lightly with sesame seeds. Bake in a preheated 375-degree oven for 15 minutes, then lower to 325 degrees and bake for 35 to 40 minutes longer. This is called all-purpose bread because we feel it has the best combination of ingredients and the texture of regular bread. It is very tasty and can be sliced thin easily. It will not crumble in the toaster and can be used for sandwiches and spreads. If for any reason you cannot use wheat germ, you can add an extra cup of soy flour or oat flour, or 1/2 cup of both instead. Makes one loaf.

SOUTHERN GRITS BREAD

1 cup soy grits
1 cup milk (preferably raw)
4 fertile eggs
¼ teaspoon sea salt
3 tablespoons butter, at room temperature

Soak the grits in the milk for 20 minutes. Beat the eggs, add the grits mixture, salt, and 2 tablespoons of the butter. Spread thinly (about 1 inch deep) in a well-oiled casserole, or pour into a cast-iron cornbread stick pan. Bake at 325 degrees for 30 minutes. Spread the top with the remaining butter. Bake until crusty and lightly browned (15 to 20 minutes). Use as a snack or supplement. Makes one loaf.

TASTY BEAN BREAD

Beans add a new dimension to making bread. This bread is sweet and dense, but not terribly heavy. It is especially delicious with apple butter. (Hypoglycemics must use apple butter *very* sparingly.)

2 cups cooked black beans or soybeans
1½ cups grain coffee, herb tea, or water
1½ cups buckwheat flour
1¼ cups whole wheat flour
¼ cup soybean flour
1 teaspoon sea salt
½ teaspoon each cinnamon, coriander, cloves
2 tablespoons butter
4 tablespoons sesame seeds

Preheat oven to 375 degrees. Puree beans in a blender with grain coffee. Add remaining ingredients and continue to knead dough for about five minutes, until it becomes slightly elastic. Oil a large bread pan (9x5x3) and, wetting your hands, shape the dough into a loaf and set in pan. Cover the pan tightly with tin foil and bake for one hour. Remove foil and bake for another 20 minutes. Let cool for one hour before cutting. Serve with fruit butter or nut butter.
Variation: Add 3 tablespoons carob powder to batter for a chocolate flavor.

GINGERBREAD

Here's a recipe for gingerbread that's dark, moist, spicy, and nutritious. Fresh carrots and oat flakes give it a chewy texture and unique flavor.

2 cups oat flakes
$1\frac{1}{2}$ pounds fresh carrots
2 inch piece of ginger root
$\frac{3}{4}$ cup chestnut flour (if none available, use $\frac{1}{2}$ cup soy flour)
$\frac{1}{2}$ cup buckwheat or rye flour
$\frac{1}{2}$ cup whole wheat pastry flour
$\frac{1}{2}$ teaspoon sea salt
2 teaspoons cinnamon
$\frac{1}{4}$ teaspoon nutmeg
1 tablespoon dry Pero (a grain coffee substitute)
1 tablespoon poppy seeds, optional
2 fertile eggs
2 cups apple juice
$\frac{1}{4}$ cup butter

Preheat oven to 375 degrees. Grate carrots either by hand or in a blender, being careful not to liquefy them. If you prefer, use cooked and mashed carrots in place of raw carrots. To prepare the ginger root, peel off the skin and finely grate the root. Squeeze out the juice and discard the stringy pulp. Combine all ingredients and mix batter thoroughly. Pour into a shallow 9x15-inch well-oiled baking dish and bake for 1 hour and 15 minutes. Serve either warm or cold. This bread is especially good served with applesauce and garnished with slivered almonds or crushed walnuts. Serves about nine.

HEALTH NUT SPONGE CAKE

1 cup whole millet
3 cups apple juice
$\frac{1}{4}$ teaspoon cloves

1 cup cooked cereal (brown rice, couscous, or oatmeal)
1½ cups whole wheat pastry flour
2 tablespoons soybean or chestnut flour
1 teaspoon sea salt
1 cup coarsely chopped nuts
2 tablespoons butter
1 lemon
¼ teaspoon nutmeg, optional
¼ teaspoon cinnamon

Rinse the millet in cold water and drain through a fine strainer. Heat a cast-iron skillet and pour in the millet. Stirring constantly, roast the millet for about 10 minutes, until it is completely dry. Add apple juice and cloves and bring to a boil; cover and simmer for 30 minutes. Preheat oven to 350 degrees. Spoon cooked millet into a large mixing bowl and mash with a fork until the grains are separated. Mash in the cooked cereal, the flours, salt, nuts, and butter. Grate the lemon over a fine grater and add the rind and juice to the batter. Mix thoroughly and pour batter into a well-oiled bread or cake pan. Sprinkle top with spices. Bake at 350 degrees for 30 minutes, then reduce temperature to 325 degrees and bake for another 50 to 60 minutes. Serves about eight.

CORN-SPOON BREAD

This light and fragrant semisweet bread holds together well and will keep moist for several days if it's wrapped and stored in the refrigerator.

3 cups whole corn meal (not degerminated or enriched)
4 cups boiling unsweetened apple juice
½ cup whole wheat pastry flour
2 cups cooked brown rice (or bulgur, cracked wheat, or millet)
¼ cup butter
3 tablespoons sesame seeds

1 teaspoon sea salt
1 fertile egg
1½ teaspoon cinnamon
¼ teaspoon coriander or nutmeg (optional)

Preheat oven to 400 degrees. Pour corn meal into a large bowl and scald with apple juice. Pour the apple juice slowly and mix the batter thoroughly to prevent lumping. Let mixture sit for 10 minutes. Add remaining ingredients, one at a time, beating well after each addition. Spoon batter into a well-oiled shallow two-quart casserole. Bake at 400 degrees the first 15 minutes, then reduce heat to 350 degrees for another 40 minutes. Serves about eight.
Variations: Chopped nuts or sunflower seeds may be added if desired.

CORN-SPOON MUFFINS

Prepare Corn-Spoon Bread. Pour into oiled muffin pans. Bake at 325 degrees for 30 to 40 minutes. For variations, add any kind of berries.

IRA G'S CORN MUFFINS

1½ cups corn meal (unprocessed)
2 cups boiling water or apple juice
1 cup cooked cereal (rice, couscous, or kasha)
2 tablespoons soybean flour
2 tablespoons arrowroot flour starch
2 tablespoons sesame seeds
½ teaspoon sea salt
2 tablespoons butter
2 fertile eggs
1 cup fresh crushed fruit (blueberries or peaches)
1 teaspoon grated lemon rind

Preheat oven to 350 degrees and insert empty muffin tins. Put corn meal into a mixing bowl and scald with water or apple juice. Stir rapidly to prevent lumping. Beat in remaining ingredients. Remove muffin tins from oven and brush well with oil. Spoon mixture to fill each well. Bake for 45 minutes.

Salad Savvy

The salad, which can be really anything, is a particularly good meal or accompaniment to a meal since it is a perfect vehicle for fresh uncooked foods. Somehow raw carrots, broccoli, cauliflower, and mushrooms look and feel out of place on a dinner plate with a portion of meat, but assume an entirely different character when they are mixed into a salad. In addition, the salad can contain sprouts, a particularly rich source of vitamins and minerals; various beans, a good source of amino acids, the building blocks of protein; and seeds and nuts. In other words, the salad is unlimited in its contents. It may be served hot or cold, as a meal in itself, or as part of a meal. It may take on an international flavor or be simply garden fresh. And most important, it supplies important complex carbohydrates, proteins, fats, vitamins, minerals, and the all-important fiber. Let your imagination run wild and make a salad.

VIM AND VIGOR SALADS
AND SALAD DRESSINGS

TUTU SALAD

1 cup finely grated carrots
1/2 cup finely chopped celery
1 cup shredded romaine
1 cup alfalfa sprouts
1/2 avocado, peeled, pitted, and mashed
lemon juice
sea salt to taste

Tutu means "grandmother" in Hawaiian, so for those who have trouble chewing, this will be helpful and healthful. In a salad bowl, combine the carrots, celery, romaine, and alfalfa sprouts. Mash the avocado with a fork or in an electric blender, adding enough lemon juice to make a thick puree. Season with salt. Pour avocado over salad and toss. Serves three to four.

ITALIAN SALAD

3 small young zucchini (about 1 pound)
3 scallions, finely chopped (optional)
2 tablespoons snipped fresh dill weed
1 tablespoon chopped parsley
1/4 teaspoon oregano
1 cup whole-milk yogurt
1 tablespoon lemon juice
1/2 cup chopped celery (optional)

Wash the zucchini and dice very finely. Place in a salad bowl with the scallions, dill, parsley, and oregano. Combine the yogurt and lemon juice and pour over zucchini. Toss to mix well. Refrigerate 30 minutes or longer before serving. Serves four to six.

MIDWEST SALAD

1 cup cooked corn kernels, cut from the cob
1 1/2 cups cottage cheese
1 tablespoon chopped green pepper
1 tablespoon chopped parsley
1 tablespoon chopped pimentos
sea salt to taste

Toss all ingredients together and store in a covered container in the refrigerator until serving time. Serves four.

DELUXE CABBAGE SLAW

1 small head green cabbage, finely shredded
1 cup shredded fresh pineapple
1 cup cashews, ground
1/4 cup water
2 tablespoons cider vinegar
sea salt to taste

Place cabbage and pineapple in a salad bowl. Mix the ground cashews with water to make a stiff paste. Add vinegar and sea salt. Pour over cabbage and pineapple and toss. Serves six to eight.

CHICKEN RING

4 envelopes unflavored gelatin
2 cans clear chicken soup
1 cup mayonnaise
1 cup celery, finely chopped
1/2 cup red pepper
1 cup green pepper, finely chopped
1 cup sliced avocado, diced
1/2 cup chopped pecans
1 1/2 cups cooked chicken, diced
4 tablespoons lemon juice
butter

Soften gelatin in cold water. Heat chicken soup and dissolve gelatin in it. Cool. When it is slightly thickened, fold in other ingredients. Pour into ring mold well greased with butter. Chill until firm. Serves four to six.

PEEK-A-BOO SALAD

8 ounces raw cottage cheese
several lettuce leaves

2 cups blueberries
watermelon
pears, halved
mint leaves

Spread lettuce leaves on plate. With small ice-cream scoop, make six watermelon balls. Cut in half. Set flat portion in center of lettuce. With large ice-cream scoop, make six balls of cottage cheese. Set each one on melon. Place half a pear on either side of cottage cheese. Fill generously with blueberries. Cut remaining pear halves into quarters. Garnish with fresh mint leaves. Serves four to six.

ALL-IN-ONE SALAD

2 cups cooked chicken or turkey, cut up into large chunks
1 cup celery cut up in $1/4$-inch slices
1 tablespoon lemon juice
sea salt to taste
dash seasoned pepper
drained cut-up unsweetened pineapple (medium-sized can)
$1/2$ cup almonds
mayonnaise to moisten (about $1/2$ cup)
lettuce leaves
3 fertile eggs, deviled and cut into quarters
1 cucumber

Mix all ingredients with mayonnaise. (See mayonnaise recipe on page 201.) Place on lettuce leaves. Garnish with deviled eggs cut in quarters and cucumber wedges. Serves six.

WALDORF SALAD

1 cup celery, diced
2 cups apples, diced
$1/2$ cup broken walnuts
2 tablespoons lemon juice
$1/4$ cup raisins

$\frac{1}{2}$ cup homemade mayonnaise
lettuce leaves

Dice the celery. Peel, core, and dice the apples and sprinkle all with lemon juice. Add raisins. Mix in mayonnaise and half of walnuts. Serve on a bed of lettuce. Sprinkle with remaining walnuts on top. Serves four to six.

COTTAGE CHEESE FRUIT SALAD

2 cups creamed cottage cheese
$1\frac{1}{2}$ cups fresh or sugarless canned fruit, diced (strawberries, pineapple, apples, peaches, plums, pears, etc.)
$\frac{1}{2}$ cup sour cream (optional)

Combine all ingredients, mix, and chill. Sprinkle with ground walnuts, sunflower seeds, or almonds. Entire recipe makes four cups.

WALDORF SALAD AU NATURAL

1 large tart apple
$\frac{1}{4}$ cup coarsely broken walnut meats
1 tablespoon fresh lemon juice
2 large ribs celery, diced
$\frac{1}{4}$ cup homemade mayonnaise
4 large lettuce leaves

Halve the apple and remove the core; do not peel. Dice the apple, sprinkle with lemon juice. Combine with the nuts and celery, and toss. Add the mayonnaise and mix well. Serve on lettuce leaves. Serves four.

ANASTASIA SALAD MOLD

2 tablespoons unflavored gelatin
1 cup water

1 cup sour cream
1 cup homemade mayonnaise
2 tablespoons lemon juice
1 teaspoon chopped fresh dill weed or $1/4$ teaspoon
   dried dill weed
1 teaspoon sea salt
1 teaspoon minced onion
1 cup chopped celery
$1/4$ cup chopped pimentos
$1/4$ cup chopped green pepper
$1/8$ teaspoon celery seed
$1/8$ teaspoon sesame seed

Sprinkle gelatin over the water to soften; cook over low heat, stirring until the gelatin is dissolved. Cool until syrupy. Fold in the remaining ingredients, stirring until evenly mixed. Pour into a mold or large bowl. Chill until firm. Turn out on plate. Serves six to eight.

EGG SALAD

6 hard-cooked fertile eggs, chilled and peeled
4 ribs celery, chopped
$1/4$ cup finely chopped onion
$1/2$ teaspoon sea salt
1 sour pickle, chopped
1 tablespoon finely minced celery tops
1 tablespoon prepared mustard
dash of freshly ground pepper
dash paprika

Chop the eggs. Combine all ingredients and mix well. Chill and serve on lettuce, or stuff three hollowed-out tomatoes. Serves three.

PINEAPPLE-LIME SALAD

1 cup pineapple packed in its own juice (unsweetened)
1 teaspoon pimento, chopped
1 teaspoon diced celery
sea salt to taste
1 tablespoon lemon juice
1 envelope unsweetened lime gelatin
½ cup hot pineapple juice (unsweetened)

Cut pineapple into cubes. Clean and dice celery and pimentos. Marinate pimentos for two hours in lemon juice and sea salt. Measure out other ingredients. Dissolve gelatin in hot water. When it begins to set, add fruit, celery, and marinated pimentos. Let stand in individual molds until set, and serve on crisp lettuce leaf. Serves four.

TROPICAL DRESSING

1 ripe avocado, peeled and pitted
1 large grapefruit, peeled and sectioned
1 large tomato, skinned
small sprig of parsley

Place the ingredients in an electric blender and blend until smooth. Yield: about 3 cups. (This dressing is for raw vegetable salads, but it can be used as a dip as well.)

TURKISH DRESSING

½ cup ground sesame seeds
sprinkle of chia seeds
1 cup yogurt or water (approximately)
juice of ½ lemon
½ clove garlic

Place seeds and one cup yogurt or water in an electric blender and blend until smooth. Add remaining ingredients and blend until smooth, adding more yogurt if necessary to give the dressing the correct consistency. Yield: about one cup. *Variation:* Add one-half cup chopped onions, one-half cup chopped celery, and one-half cup mixed alfalfa, mung bean, and lentil sprouts. Blend until smooth for a mock tuna sandwich spread or dip.

FAMILY DRESSING

1 cup cottage cheese
1 tablespoon lemon juice
$1/4$ cup tomato juice, approximately
1 hard-cooked egg, chopped
1 teaspoon prepared mustard

Put the cottage cheese and lemon juice and mustard in an electric blender. Add $1/4$ cup tomato juice and blend until very smooth, adding more tomato juice if necessary. Stir the egg into the dressing just before using. Makes about one cup.

DOWN EAST DRESSING

1 cup buttermilk
1 teaspoon frozen apple juice (concentrate)
1 teaspoon lemon juice
1 teaspoon dried onion flakes
1 teaspoon dill weed
1 teaspoon chia seed
pepper and allspice, to taste

Mix together all ingredients. Season to taste with pepper and ground allspice. Chill before serving.

EXOTIC DRESSING

3 tablespoons ground sesame seeds
3 tablespoons tamari (soy sauce)
raw milk

Mix ground sesame seeds and tamari together with enough milk to make the correct consistency for a salad dressing. Makes about $\frac{1}{3}$ cup.

FEZ DRESSING

Mix equal parts of cottage cheese and yogurt with 1 teaspoon dill weed. Chill.

AEGEAN DRESSING

1 ripe avocado, peeled, pitted, and mashed or pureed
1 cup yogurt
1 tablespoon tamari (soy sauce)
$\frac{1}{8}$ teaspoon oregano
1 tablespoon lemon juice
1 tablespoon chopped onion

Combine all ingredients and mix well. Makes about $2\frac{1}{2}$ cups. This dressing is good served over tossed green salads garnished with sprouts.

DRESSING A LA RUSSE

$\frac{3}{4}$ cup tomato juice
$\frac{1}{2}$ cup buttermilk
1 teaspoon lemon juice
$\frac{1}{8}$ teaspoon dry mustard
dash dehydrated onion flakes
sea salt
1 medium dill pickle, diced fine

Simmer tomato juice until reduced to half volume. In blender, combine all ingredients except dill pickle and blend well. Add diced dill pickle; blend. Serves two.

HEAVY DRESSING

2 teaspoons unflavored gelatin
2 tablespoons cold water
2 teaspoons dehydrated onion flakes
$1/4$ cup lemon juice
1 teaspoon sea salt
1 teaspoon dry mustard
$1/8$ teaspoon black pepper
1 cup buttermilk
1 teaspoon chia seed

Soften gelatin in cold water in small saucepan. Stir in onion flakes, lemon juice, sea salt, mustard, and pepper. Heat, stirring to dissolve gelatin. Add buttermilk and chia seeds. Refrigerate until set. Whip in a mixer or blender before serving. Serves four. (Use as salad dressing just as you would use mayonnaise for cole slaw, to bind chopped foods, etc.)

JACK'S FAVORITE SALAD DRESSING

8 ounces tomato sauce
3 tablespoons lemon juice
1 teaspoon Worcestershire sauce
1 tablespoon tamari sauce (optional)
$1/2$ teaspoon dried dill weed
$1/2$ teaspoon dried basil, crushed
1 teaspoon onion, diced
2 cloves garlic (minced)
1 1" long chili pepper (ground)

Put all ingredients in blender and blend until smooth.

MARCELLA'S SOUR CREAM

Put some crumbled hoop cheese (this cheese is suited especially well to hypoglycemics) into blender. Blend with sufficient liquid (buttermilk, milk) to achieve consistency of sour cream. Use on salads, baked potatoes, etc. (Hoop cheese is sometimes called farmer cheese, baker's cheese, and pot cheese.)

ALL-STAR SALAD DRESSING AND
SALAD IDEAS

Into salad bowl put the following:

1 teaspoon garlic salt (or garlic clove, crushed with a little sea salt)
$1/2$ teaspoon dry mustard
$1/2$ teaspoon oregano (whole leaf)
$1/2$ teaspoon basil (whole leaf)
$1/2$ teaspoon marjoram (whole leaf),
$1/2$ teaspoon thyme (whole leaf)
$1/8$ teaspoon dill weed (optional)
$1/8$ teaspoon pepper (optional)

Stir.

Add:

$1 1/2$ tablespoons olive oil
$3/4$ tablespoon lemon juice
2 dashes Worcestershire sauce

Stir.

(If you would like a cheese dressing, add 1 tablespoon blue cheese and mash into dressing.)
Add all your cut vegetables, and toss.
Add a complete protein, either 4 ounces cottage cheese or natural cheese; hard-boiled eggs; meat; chicken; fish or other seafood.
Top your salad with alfalfa sprouts. Serves two to three.

TASTY HEALTH MAYONNAISE

1 large fertile egg
$1/2$ teaspoon sea salt
$1/4$ teaspoon paprika
3 tablespoons lemon juice
$1/2$ teaspoon dry mustard
1 cup vegetable oil (preferably olive oil)

In the blender, combine all ingredients except the oil. Make sure the oil is very fresh. Blend on low until mixed. With the blender running on medium, begin adding the oil very slowly, one drop at a time, then in a steady drip; as the mixture begins to thicken, stir slightly with a rubber spatula so that it will not stop moving. Continue dripping and blending until the mixture is the thickness of mayonnaise. Remember, the mayonnaise is going to be getting thicker as you add more oil, not thinner. Don't panic if it doesn't seem to be getting thick. If the mayonnaise is still not thick enough for your taste after all the oil has been added, add a small amount of oil, remembering to continue blending. Store mayonnaise in the refrigerator. Makes $1/4$ cups.

Energy-maintainer Snacks

Frequent snacks are as much a part of the successful treatment of hypoglycemia as the warning not to eat sugar. The following are some examples of how you can vary snacks.

It is a good idea to keep on hand at all times "emergency" foods such as seeds, nuts and grains, canned tuna, salmon, and sardines.

Cheese for snacks should not be restricted in variety. Use Jack, cheddar, pot, farmer, and cottage cheese, but always unprocessed ones. Be wary only of cheese spreads as they usually are mixed with corn starch and other refined carbohydrates and additives.

APPLE, CHEESE, AND SOYBEAN BALLS

$1/2$ cup sharp cheddar, grated
$1/2$ cup apple, peeled and grated
$1/2$ cup crushed soybeans
$1/4$ cup sesame seeds

Mix apple and cheese together. Form into balls with tea-spoon. Roll in crushed soybeans and sesame seeds. Set in refrigerator to chill. Pierce with toothpicks and serve. Makes 10 to 12 balls.

PEANUT BUTTER WITH CHOPPED APPLE

Mix the following: 2 level teaspoons peanut butter, 1 heaping teaspoon grated apple with the peel, 2 ounces of milk mixed with 2 ounces of water. Spread on toast or use as a filler for celery.

PEANUT BUTTER NUT BALLS

Mix 1 heaping teaspoon peanut butter with $1/8$ teaspoon grated apple. Separate and pat into four balls. Sprinkle with chopped pecans, and refrigerate. Have two balls for a mid-morning snack with 4 ounces milk. Make a dozen and serve with beverages.

STUFFED CELERY

Mix 1 ounce plain yogurt with 1 ounce Swiss cheese and 1 tablespoon shelled and chopped pistachio nuts. Stuff celery with mixture. Enjoy with any whole fruit.

YOGURT WITH FRUIT

Put whole-milk plain yogurt in blender with 1 cup mashed raspberries, blackberries, or blueberries to taste. Blend on chop and then on frappe for at least 5 minutes. Pour into tall, thin glass.

BEEF BOUILLON SNACK

A when-you-are-not-hungry suggestion: 6 ounces hot beef bouillon topped with 1/2 crumbled brown rice wafer.

Other Quick Snacks

A good-sized handful of nuts
1/2 brown rice wafer spread with tuna, with 4 ounces milk
Fresh sliced apple spread with peanut butter
Mixture of any seeds and nuts

Mid-morning Snack

Shrimp cocktail (1 ounce)
Any unsweetened fruit juice, or better yet, eat the whole fruit
Or reheated whole-grain cereal left over from breakfast

Mid-afternoon Snack

Jack cheese (1 ounce) on brown rice wafers
Whole fresh tomato

Nighttime Snack

Sandman Soda (4 large strawberries, or other fruit in season, blended with 1/2 cup raw milk)
1 ounce cottage cheese with chopped vegetables or small amounts of any fresh or unsweetened fruit or nuts and seeds

GRILLED TOMATO SNACK

Lightly dust slices of tomato with oregano, bread with small amount of wheat germ and parmesan cheese, and grill under moderate flame until hot.

PARTY EGG SPREAD

8 hard-cooked fertile eggs, diced or sieved
1½ cups sour cream
2 teaspoon finely chopped onion
¼ cup chopped parsley
2 teaspoon lemon juice
1 teaspoon sea salt
¼ teaspoon cayenne pepper
3 drops tabasco sauce

In a bowl, combine all ingredients. Beat until smooth. Refrigerate until ready to spread on slices of any whole-grain bread. Makes about 3 cups.

WORK-OF-ART DOLLOPS

1½ pounds peanut butter
2 cups carob powder (unsweetened)
2 tablespoons cinnamon
1 teaspoon nutmeg
½ cup dry milk powder (optional)
2 cups chopped walnuts
1 cup whole raw milk (or more if needed)

Mix dry ingredients together well. Add remaining ingredients. Form into balls about the size of a ping-pong ball or smaller. Do not cook. Eat as is. Also good frozen. Finger-licking good!

BANANA DRINK

1 cup milk (preferably raw)
1 fertile egg*
$1/2$ banana
$1/4$ teaspoon vanilla extract
1 teaspoon protein powder

In a blender, combine all ingredients and blend until smooth. Serve cold. Serves one.
* Raw eggs should not be used frequently because a chemical in the raw egg white destroys biotin. You may coddle the egg for this drink by cracking it into hot water and allowing it to set slightly. If you use just the yolk you needn't cook it.

ORANGE DRINK

$1/2$ cup milk (preferably raw)
1 fertile egg (coddled) or raw yolk
$1/2$ cup orange juice
1 teaspoon protein powder

In a blender, combine all ingredients. Blend until smooth. Serve cold. Serves one.

MAPLE-FLAVORED DRINK

1 cup milk, chilled
1 fertile egg (coddled) or raw yolk
1 teaspoon instant decaffeinated coffee granules or Pero
1 teaspoon maple-flavored extract

In a blender, combine all ingredients and blend until frothy. Serve immediately. Serves one.

PROTEIN DRINK

1 cup raw milk, chilled
1 fertile egg (coddled)

1 teaspoon vanilla

1 teaspoon protein powder (store powder in refrigerator when not in use; tastes better when cold)

1/4 teaspoon Dr. Bronner's Barleymalt Sweetener, Stevia, or Sucanat

Mix together all ingredients in a blender. Half can be used between each meal or all at once in place of breakfast.

HOLIDAY EGGNOG

3 fertile eggs, separated
2 tablespoons barley malt extract
4 cups chilled soy milk or fresh whole raw milk
2 teaspoons vanilla extract
3 teaspoons cinnamon
nutmeg

Beat the egg whites until stiff; beat the yolks in a blender or by hand until foamy. Add barley malt to the yolks and beat again. Add soy or raw whole milk and vanilla. Fold in egg whites. Flavor with nutmeg and cinnamon. Serve cold. Makes about four 9-ounce servings.

COTTAGE CHEESE TOMATO COCKTAIL

1 cup tomato juice
1/2 cup cottage cheese
dash sea salt
dash onion powder
dash celery salt
dash tabasco sauce (optional)

Put all ingredients in blender and blend until smooth.

CAFE D'HERBE

For a beverage treat loaded with health-giving goodness, steep fresh or dried Comfrey and mint herbs. Then add Pero or other coffee substitute to taste. May be served with or without milk or cream. On a hot day, serve as a cold drink.

CAPPUCCINO FOR THE AWARE

Add hot water to any decaffeinated coffee, Pero, Pionier, or Cafix grain coffee substitute. Shake in a generous amount of cinnamon to taste. Add whole raw milk or cream. Nutmeg may also be added if desired. Your whole family will enjoy this hearty, warming drink.

Janet Delmonte's RECOVERY SOUP

We give this a 5 star rating! This dear friend of mine gives this delicious and nutritious soup instead of flowers, at times of physical or emotional crisis. (We were Girl Scout leaders together years ago, and even then we didn't encourage them to sell those sugar cookies!)

$1\frac{1}{2}$ pounds ground beef
2 large onions, diced
2 large cloves garlic, minced fine (or $\frac{1}{2}$ teaspoon garlic powder)
$\frac{1}{2}$ large green pepper, diced
3 stalks celery, diced
1 large can tomato juice (46 ounces)
2 cups water
1 large potato, peeled and diced
2 cups coarsely cut cabbage
1 large package (20 ounces) frozen mixed vegetables (carrots, peas, green beans, corn, and lima beans)
1 can (15 ounces) either garbanzo or kidney beans
2 tablespoons Schilling's Italian seasoning (marjoram, thyme, rosemary, savory, sage, oregano, and sweet basil combined)
1 tablespoon dried parsley (or $\frac{1}{4}$ cup fresh chopped parsley)

1 tablespoon tamari (soy sauce)
3/4 teaspoon ground black pepper (or to taste)

Sauté beef in enough oil to just grease the bottom of a
5-quart pot. Add onion and garlic, and stir to crumble beef.
When beef loses its pink color and onions are transparent,
thoroughly drain off all fat. Then add all the remaining
ingredients, in order given. Bring to a boil, stirring very
frequently to avoid burning the bottom. Reduce heat to low,
and let simmer about a half-hour, stirring frequently. (Can
be thickened with a mixture of 1/3 cup soy flour mixed with
2/3 cup water, if desired.) Also can add more water to obtain
desired consistency. SOUP IS VERY THICK.
NOTE: If using food processor, use slicer, NOT SHREDDER
(or vegetables will sink to bottom and burn easily!)

Entrees To Health—Meat, Fish, and Fowl

PARTICIPATION BEEF

1 1/2 pounds lean round steak
garlic powder to taste
dash of freshly ground pepper
butter as needed
sea salt to taste

This is fine with round steak, but if you prefer, use a better
cut. Remove all fat and gristle from the meat and cut into
bite-sized cubes. Dust lightly with garlic powder and pepper.
Fill a small saucepan or fondue pot with butter and heat
until bubbling. Have fun while each person skewers a cube
of beef and dips it into the hot butter for one minute to
cook. Salt to taste and eat immediately. Repeat until all the
beef has been eaten. Serve with chili sauce, ketchup, and
other sauces. Nice as an hors d'oeuvre.

VEGETABLE CHILI BEANS

1 can cooked soybeans
1 small can tomato puree
$1/4$ teaspoon sea salt
$1/4$ teaspoon chili powder
dash of garlic powder
1 tablespoon onion
$1/4$ teaspoon freshly ground pepper
1 tablespoon butter (preferably raw)
$1/2$ teaspoon cumin seed
1 tablespoon bran

Combine all ingredients in a saucepan. Bring to a slow boil, then simmer, stirring occasionally, for 30 minutes, or until the sauce is thick. Ground meat can be added if desired.

HAWAIIAN CHICKEN

1 3-pound fryer chicken
1 cup water
2 tablespoons butter
3 scallions, finely sliced
$1/2$ cup diced celery
$1/4$ teaspoon cayenne pepper
small can water chestnuts
3 tablespoons tamari soy sauce
$3/4$ cup whole almonds
$1/2$ medium green pepper, diced
1 cup fresh pineapple chunks (ripe)
1 teaspoon sea salt
1 can bean sprouts, freshened with cold water, or fresh
   sprouts

Place the chicken on a rack in a pressure cooker or steamer. Add the water, cover, and pressure-cook or steam until tender (about 15 minutes). Remove the chicken and discard the bones and skin. In a large skillet, heat the butter and sauté the scallions, celery, and pepper until softened. Add the boned chicken, the water in which it was cooked, and the rest of the ingredients except the bean sprouts (unless they are fresh and raw). Cover and simmer gently 10 minutes. Remove the cover and simmer 10 minutes longer. Heat the bean sprouts and water chestnuts in a little water, drain, and squeeze out the excess moisture. Pour the chicken mixture over the hot sprouts and serve.

PEPPERS A POULE

Basic White Sauce (see following recipe)
2 cups diced cold chicken
1 small onion, chopped, or leeks
3 or 4 black olives, sliced
¾ cup chopped celery
sea salt and pepper to taste
pinch of dried parsley
6 medium green peppers, cored
1 cup chicken broth made with sea salt

Prepare the sauce, then blend it in the blender until smooth. Combine the chicken, vegetables, olives, and sauce in a bowl, mixing well. Season to taste. Stuff the mixture into the peppers. Place in a small buttered casserole. Pour the chicken broth around the peppers. Bake at 350 degrees for 1 hour.

BASIC WHITE SAUCE

2 tablespoons butter
2 tablespoons soy flour
1 cup half and half
fertile egg yolk, beaten
dash of white pepper
sea salt to taste

Melt the butter in the top of a double boiler. Blend in the soy flour, mixing to a paste. Add half and half slowly, stirring with a whisk to avoid lumps. Add the egg yolk and seasonings, and heat, stirring frequently. Do not boil. Continue cooking until the desired thickness is reached. If necessary, thin with milk.

Seafood

BAKED FILLET OF SOLE

1 pound fillet of sole (or flounder, cod, haddock, etc.)
2 tablespoons butter
$1/2$ teaspoon parsley flakes
1 teaspoon sesame seeds
$1/4$ teaspoon freshly ground pepper
dash of paprika
dash of thyme
1 teaspoon wheat germ
sea salt

Place the fillets in a well-buttered baking dish and dot with the raw butter. Crush the parsley and sprinkle over the fish, along with the other ingredients, except the sea salt. Place in a preheated 375-degree oven and bake for 25 to 30 minutes, or until the fish is opaque and flakes easily. Remove from the oven and salt to taste just before serving.

BROILED FISH FILLETS

1 pound fish fillets or 2 pounds whole fish, cleaned and
    trimmed
$1/4$ cup melted butter
paprika
dash of onion powder
sprinkle of garlic powder
freshly ground pepper

sea salt to taste
$\frac{1}{2}$ lemon, sliced

Place the fish on a buttered broiler rack over a broiler pan. Brush generously with melted butter and sprinkle with paprika, onion powder, and garlic powder. Place in the broiler 5 or 6 inches from the heat. Broil 3 minutes for fillets, 5 for the whole fish. Turn, season with paprika, onion powder, and pepper on the other side. Continue broiling until the fish flakes easily (1 or 2 minutes for fillets, 3 minutes for whole fish). If you find the odor of fish unpleasant, try removing the skin before broiling, and broil 6 to 8 inches from the heat. This eliminates most of the fat and the "fishy" smell. Salt to taste and serve with lemon slices.

BAKED HALIBUT TARRAGON

$\frac{1}{4}$ cup melted butter
1 teaspoon dry mustard
1 teaspoon tarragon
1 large halibut steak (about $1\frac{1}{2}$ pounds) or any other fish
  steak
dash of thyme

Melt the butter and mix in the spices. Arrange the fish in a large, shallow baking dish. Pour or brush the butter sauce over the fish. Bake at 375 degrees for about 25 minutes, or until the fish flakes easily with a fork.

COD AU GRATIN

$1\frac{1}{2}$ pounds cod fillets
1 leek or 2 scallions, sliced thin
2 ounces butter
$1\frac{1}{2}$ cups milk (preferably raw)
dash of paprika
$\frac{1}{2}$ teaspoon sea salt

½ cup grated cheese (preferably Gruyere or any unprocessed cheese)
dash of oregano
½ lemon, sliced

Place the cod fillets in a single layer in a greased casserole and set aside. In a small saucepan, melt the butter and cook the leek or scallions for 5 minutes on very low heat. Pour over the fish and add the milk and seasonings. Cover the casserole and bake at 375 degrees until the fish flakes easily (about 20 minutes). Uncover and sprinkle with the grated cheese. Bake in the oven at 425 degrees until the cheese is melted and browned (10 minutes). Serve with lemon slices.

FISH BURGERS

½ cup water
1 cup frozen sliced carrots
1 pound white fish fillets (sole, flounder, cod, etc.)
2 extra large fertile eggs
½ cup cream
¼ cup soy flour
1 tablespoon butter (preferably raw)
1 tablespoon minced onion
¼ teaspoon sage
½ teaspoon sea salt
dash of nutmeg
dash of freshly ground pepper
1 thick slice homemade oatmeal bread, crumbled fine in the blender
butter as needed
lemon slices

Heat the water and cook the carrots, covered, until soft enough to mash. Remove the carrots and set aside. Add a little more water to the pan if needed and cook the fish, covered, for 5 minutes, or until the fish can be flaked with a fork. Set aside. In the blender, combine the eggs, cream, flour, butter, and seasonings. Blend and add to the cooked fish. Add the carrots and half the bread crumbs. Mash the entire mixture well with a fork, until thoroughly mixed. Chill until the mixture is fairly stiff. Form into patties or croquettes of the desired shape. Roll carefully in the rest of the bread crumbs. Fry in $1/4$ inch of butter on low heat until evenly browned. Serve with lemon slices.

SALMON PATTIES

$2^{1/2}$ slices homemade oatmeal bread
1 medium onion, quartered
1-pound can red salmon
dash of freshly ground pepper
dash of oregano
2 fertile eggs
$1/2$ teaspoon paprika
$1/2$ teaspoon sea salt
butter as needed

Make the bread into crumbs in the blender and transfer to a large bowl. Blend the eggs and onion in the blender by turning it on and off until the onion is grated but not liquefied. Pour the mixture into the bowl with the crumbs. Flake the salmon with a fork and add to the onion mixture. Season and mix well. Heat butter in a frying pan. When the butter is mildly hot, place the patties in the pan. Heat until evenly browned.

Desserts With A Purpose

These desserts contain no sugar, honey, or artificial sweeteners, and are the only kind anyone should eat, for by changing the quality of the carbohydrates you eat, you can change the quality of your health and life.

Each person with hypoglycemia has a different tolerance for carbohydrates. Furthermore, an individual's tolerance fluctuates from time to time, depending on the stress he is experiencing. Under stress, emotional or physical, the hypoglycemic's tolerance for carbohydrates is low.

Many of the following recipes have a larger amount of natural fructose (fruit sugar) than some hypoglycemics can tolerate. Therefore, if you are a hypoglycemic:

1. Try these recipes only when you are feeling well and relatively stress-free;

2. keep the portions small; and

3. do not eat these desserts more than twice a week, and be sure to leave three to four days between eating them, to test your tolerance for the increased amounts of high-quality carbohydrates found in these recipes.

These recipes should be tried only during the detective stage, *not* during the first, second, and third stages of treatment.

These desserts are nutritious and can be used regularly by non-hypoglycemics, and they are much less fattening than desserts made with poor-quality carbohydrates.

HOLIDAY CAKE

This spicy orange-colored cake is delicious.

1 pound carrots, grated
1/2 cup chestnut flour or pureed chestnuts
2 tablespoons soybean flour
1/2 cup flour (brown rice, barley, or whole wheat pastry flour)
1 cup cooked grain (any cereal)
2 fertile eggs
1/4 cup butter

1½ cups liquid (grain coffee or fruit juice)
½ teaspoon each: sea salt, ground cloves
1 teaspoon ground ginger
¼ teaspoon nutmeg

Preheat oven to 350 degrees. Mix all ingredients well. Pour batter into an oiled casserole or shallow cake pan and cover. Bake for 30 minutes, remove cover, and bake for another 20 to 30 minutes.
Variations: This cake can also be steamed in a pressure cooker. Place pan on a rack, with 2 inches of water around the pan. Bring up to full pressure. Lower flame and cook with medium pressure for 1 hour and 15 minutes. Let pressure fall normally. Add ½ cup raisins or currants or Dr. Bronner's Barleymalt Sweetner for a sweeter flavor.

AMSTERDAM TORTE

1 cup whole wheat pastry flour
¼ cup chestnut flour or soybean flour
¾ cup barley or oat flour
2 teaspoons cinnamon
¼ teaspoon sea salt
1 teaspoon vanilla extract
¼ teaspoon allspice
¼ teaspoon cloves
1 cup apple juice or apple cider
3 fertile eggs, separated
¼ cup sesame or safflower oil
2 tablespoons sesame butter or almond butter
4 large apples, cored and thinly sliced
¼ cup crushed nuts

Preheat oven to 350 degrees. Sift dry ingredients, except nuts, into a bowl. Mix in oil and set aside. Mix apple juice and vanilla. Beat egg yolks until foamy. Beat the whites until they form soft peaks. Add apple juice and sesame butter to batter and beat until smooth. Beat in egg yolks and fold in egg whites. Oil a 9x12-inch cake pan. Pour in half the batter and arrange a layer of apple slices on top. Repeat and cover with crushed nuts. Bake for 1 hour.

BORODENKO'S POLISH CAKE

2 cups cooked and mashed soybeans
1 cup buckwheat flour
1 cup brown rice flour
3 apples, grated, or 1 cup applesauce
1 cup apple juice
$\frac{1}{2}$ cup ground dried fruit
$\frac{1}{2}$ teaspoon sea salt
1 teaspoon grated lemon rind
2 tablespoons sesame seeds
2 tablespoons oil
2 fertile eggs

Preheat oven to 350 degrees. Beat all ingredients together and pour into an oiled 9x12-inch cake pan. Bake for 1 hour, or until top is firm and a toothpick inserted in the center comes out clean.

Variations: Add 1 teaspoon cinnamon and a dash of nutmeg. Chopped nuts or $\frac{1}{4}$ cup sesame butter or almond butter can be added to batter for a richer cake. Or add 3 table-spoons carob powder for a chocolate flavor. Serves eight.

"INCREDIBLE" CAKE

Parsnips become incredibly sweet when cooked for a long time, and in this cake they resemble bananas in taste and texture.

3 pounds parsnips
2 tablespoons butter
1 teaspoon sea salt
4 cups apple juice

1 lemon
1 teaspoon vanilla extract
1½ cups couscous
¼ cup nut butter
½ cup nuts
¼ teaspoon ginger
¼ teaspoon nutmeg

Scrub parsnips in cold water and slice into thin, round pieces. Heat butter in large skillet and saute parsnips for 10 minutes. Add sea salt and 1 cup apple juice. Cover and cook for 45 minutes. Puree parsnips. Preheat oven to 375 degrees. Add remaining apple juice to parsnips and simmer in a covered pan for 10 minutes. Grate the lemon rind and add to the parsnip mixture along with lemon juice and vanilla. Mix in couscous and nut butter and nuts, add ginger and nutmeg and transfer to an oiled casserole. Bake for 1 hour. Serves eight to ten.

WOJCIK'S POLISH COOKIES

1½ cups barley flour
½ cup buckwheat flour
½ cup chestnut flour or sweet rice flour
½ cup roasted sesame seeds
¼ teaspoon sea salt
2 tablespoons butter
1½ cups apple juice
1 fertile egg, beaten
1 teaspoon cinnamon
½ teaspoon nutmeg

Mix flours, seeds, and sea salt together. Add butter, rubbing it into the dough with your fingers to make a mealy consistency. Add liquid and egg, a small amount at a time. As soon as the dough becomes soft and holds together, stop adding the liquid and knead for about 5 minutes. Then pinch off pieces of dough and roll into 1-inch balls. Brush cookie sheet with oil and press dough onto surface with the tines of a moistened fork. Flatten out each ball to a 2-inch diameter. Sprinkle with cinnamon and nutmeg. Bake for 20 minutes.

VITA "C" DELIGHTS

1 tablespoon bran flakes
3 cups sweet brown rice flour or regular brown rice flour
1/4 cup Sucanat
1/2 teaspoon sea salt
1/4 cup butter
1/4 cup roasted sesame seeds
1 apple, grated
1 lemon (use all the grated rind and peel)
1 fertile egg

Preheat oven to 350 degrees and insert cookie sheets. Mix all ingredients together. Roll dough into small balls. Remove cookie sheets and brush with oil. Press dough onto sheets and press down with the tines of a wet fork until diameter is about 21/2 inches and dough is 1/8 inch thick. Bake for 10 minutes, then turn cookies over with a spatula and bake for another 5 minutes.

MOTHER EARTH COOKIES

1 cup cooked cracked wheat or bulgur
1 cup whole wheat pastry flour
1/2 cup rye flour or buckwheat flour
1/4 cup soybean flour or chestnut flour
1/4 cup chopped nuts or sunflower seeds
1/4 cup butter
3/4 cup fruit juice
11/2 teaspoon cinnamon
1/2 teaspoon coriander

$1/2$ teaspoon sea salt
2 fertile eggs

Preheat oven to 350 degrees. Mix all ingredients well in a large bowl. Knead for a few minutes. Form dough into small balls. Place balls on an oiled cookie sheet and press down with a wet fork. The thinner the dough, the crisper the cookies will be. Bake for 15 to 20 minutes. These cookies are light and crunchy. The top may be glazed with fruit butter during the last 5 minutes of baking for a sweeter cookie.

LYNETTE'S PEANUT BUTTER WAFERS

3 cups wheat bran or rice bran
$1^{1/2}$ cups natural peanut butter (not hydrogenated and with no additives)
1 fertile egg
1 cup cooked grain (rice, couscous, or oatmeal or any cooked whole grain)
1 teaspoon cinnamon
1 tablespoon dry Pero (a grain coffee substitute)
$1/4$ teaspoon nutmeg

Preheat oven to 375 degrees. Pour the bran into a mixing bowl. Using a wooden spoon or rubber spatula, work the peanut butter into the bran and add other ingredients, mixing thoroughly. Dough should be fairly stiff but easy to knead. Wetting your hands frequently with cold water, pinch off pieces of dough and roll into balls 1 inch in diameter. Oil a cookie sheet and place balls 3 inches apart. Using a moistened fork, make a crisscross pattern by pressing the tines deeply into the dough. Bake for about 12 minutes.

WHOLE-WHEAT SNAPPERS

These are crisp and can be used with dips or spreads or for snacks.

2 cups cooked cracked wheat or any other cracked cereal
1 cup whole wheat pastry flour
$1/2$ cup corn flour or millet flour
2 tablespoons soybean flour
$1/2$ teaspoon sea salt
2 teaspoons cinnamon or coriander
3 tablespoons sesame or poppy seeds
2 tablespoons bran flakes
caraway seeds (optional)

Preheat oven to 400 degrees. Knead all ingredients together except seeds. Dough should be firm, but if it's too stiff, add a little water. Dough can either be rolled out on a well-floured bread board and cut into triangles, circles, etc., or rolled out directly on an oiled cookie sheet. Score the sheet with a wet knife and sprinkle dough with seeds. Prick tiny holes in crackers with a fork to allow steam to escape. Bake for 15 minutes.

Pastries

For best results in making flaky doughs, chill the oil and use very cold water. Don't knead the dough too much—excess kneading brings out the gluten, which can make a pastry dough very tough.

OAK-FLAKE PIECRUST

$1/2$ cup oat flakes
$3/4$ cup brown rice flour
$1/2$ teaspoon sea salt
$1/3$ cup oil
1 fertile egg
$1/2$ teaspoon cinnamon
2-3 tablespoons cold water or fruit juice
2 tablespoons crushed nuts or seeds

Mix together oat flakes, rice flour, salt, oil, and cinnamon. Add nuts or seeds. Dough should be very crumbly. Add egg and a small amount of water. As soon as dough begins to hold together, stop adding water. Dough will be very soft and doesn't need to be rolled out. For a bottom crust, simply press dough into a pie pan with your fingers. For a top crust, crumble over pie filling. Use leftover crust as a cookie dough by adding chopped nuts or fruit and bake at the same time as you make the pie.

WHOLE-WHEAT PIECRUST

1 cup whole wheat pastry flour
1 cup whole wheat flour
$1/4$ teaspoon sea salt
$1/3$ cup cold oil
$1/2$ teaspoon cinnamon
$1/2$ tablespoon grated lemon or orange rind
$1/3$ cup ice water
2 tablespoons crushed nuts or seeds
1 fertile egg

Combine flours and salt in a mixing bowl. Add oil and mix with your fingers or a fork until mixture resembles fine meal. Add remaining ingredients and knead gently, just until mixture begins to form a ball. Pie dough should be somewhat flaky for best results. Roll dough out on a floured board and transfer to pie pan.

THREE-GRAIN PIECRUST

$1/2$ cup buckwheat flour
$1/2$ cup brown rice flour
$1/4$ cup whole wheat pastry flour
2 tablespoons crushed seeds or nuts
$1/2$ teaspoon sea salt
$1/2$ teaspoon cinnamon

$\frac{1}{3}$ cup butter
few tablespoons cold water

Preheat oven to 375 degrees. Combine dry ingredients in a bowl and rub butter into flours with your fingers. Add just enough water so that dough holds together, but it should remain crumbly. Press into a 9-inch pie pan and bake for 15 minutes. The beauty of this simple pie dough is that it resembles a graham cracker crust and it doesn't have to be rolled out! It holds up especially well under creamy fillings and puddings. Or you can use it as a topping for fruit desserts by simply crumbling cooked pie dough over applesauce, fresh or dried stewed fruit, etc.

CORN MEAL PIECRUST

$\frac{1}{2}$ cup corn flour
$\frac{1}{2}$ cup boiling water
$\frac{1}{3}$ cup butter
$\frac{1}{4}$ teaspoon sea salt
$1\frac{1}{2}$ cups whole wheat pastry flour
1 fertile egg

Scald the corn flour with boiling water. Add oil and beat with a fork for a few minutes to blend. Add salt and flour. Beat in egg. Refrigerate dough for a few minutes before rolling. Good with squash or pumpkin pie filling.

COUNTRY PIECRUST

$1\frac{1}{2}$ cups rye flour
$2\frac{1}{2}$ cups whole wheat pastry flour
$\frac{3}{4}$ cup oil
$\frac{1}{2}$ teaspoon sea salt
1 tablespoon poppy seeds
$\frac{1}{3}$ cup ice water

Combine all ingredients except water until fine and crumbly. Add water gradually and stop when dough begins to pull away from sides of bowl. Knead gently and roll out on a well-floured board.

YANKEE COBBLER

1 tablespoon bran flakes
1 cup oatmeal
1/2 teaspoon baking soda
1/3 cup butter
1/3 cup water
11/2 teaspoon grated lemon rind
5 sweet apples, peeled and cut into eighths
2 teaspoon cinnamon
1/2 teaspoon nutmeg
2 teaspoon lemon juice
1/2 teaspoon ground ginger

Preheat oven to 375 degrees. In a bowl, combine bran, oatmeal, and baking soda. Gradually cut in butter until mixture is crumbly. Add water and lemon rind. Work mixture into a paste. Arrange apples in a buttered baking dish. Sprinkle with cinnamon, nutmeg, lemon juice, and ginger. Spread the oatmeal paste over the apples. Bake for about 45 minutes or until pastry is well browned.

Puddings And Custards

BAKED CUSTARD

1/2 cup whole milk
1 fertile egg
1/8 teaspoon almond extract or vanilla
dash nutmeg and cinnamon

Scald milk. Beat egg slightly. Add scalded milk to egg and mix well. Add extract. Pour into custard cup that has been rinsed in cold water, and bake in 325 degree oven for 45 minutes. Results are better if custard is baked with cup surrounded by water. When a pointed knife inserted in custard emerges clean, it is done. Do not hesitate to prolong baking time for browner custard. Vanilla, lemon, or maple may be used instead of the almond extract. If a sweeter custard can be tolerated, add $1/4$ teaspoon barley malt extract.

Easy To Prepare
Fruit and Vegetable
Desserts

SPICED PEARS

6 large pears
$1/2$ teaspoon sea salt
1 cup apple or orange juice
1 heaping tablespoon arrowroot flour starch
$1/4$ teaspoon nutmeg
$1/4$ teaspoon ground ginger
$1/4$ teaspoon cinnamon

Preheat oven to 350 degrees. Wash pears thoroughly in cold water and cut in half lengthwise. Place pears in a baking dish and sprinkle with sea salt. Pour in juice and cover pan. Bake for 30 minutes. Remove cover and drain off cooking liquid. Mix reserved liquid with arrowroot starch. Return sauce to pan and sprinkle pears with nutmeg, cinnamon, and ginger. Cover pan and bake for another 15 to 20 minutes, basting fruit occasionally with glaze.

BUNNY PUDDING

2 pounds fresh carrots
1 tablespoon butter
2 cups liquid (herbal tea or fruit juice)
2 tablespoons arrowroot flour starch
1/2 cup pureed chestnuts
1/2 teaspoon sea salt
1 1/2 teaspoons cinnamon
1/2 teaspoon nutmeg

Slice carrots diagonally into thin, round pieces. To the carrots, add 1 cup liquid and butter, cover pan, and simmer for 30 minutes. Drain carrots, reserving cooking liquid, and puree in a food mill. Return liquid to pan, stir arrowroot until dissolved, then add remaining liquid, pureed carrots, chestnuts, sea salt, and spices. Simmer for 10 minutes or until very thick. Pudding may also be poured into a casserole and baked for 20 minutes at 375 degrees.

GUEST APPLES

4-5 large tart red apples
2 1/2 cups apple or orange juice
1 1/2 teaspoon cinnamon
1/2 teaspoon sea salt
1 tablespoon dry Pero (grain coffee substitute)
1 heaping tablespoon arrowroot flour starch

Wash apples thoroughly. Cut into thin, round pieces. Bring 2 cups of the juice to a boil in a deep saucepan or skillet. Add cinnamon and sea salt and then boil several apple rings at a time for 3 to 5 minutes. Remove cooked apples with a slotted spoon and repeat process until all fruit is cooked. Dilute Pero and arrowroot with remaining juice. Mix well and add to cooking liquid. Simmer, stirring constantly until mixture becomes thick. Pour glaze over apples and serve warm or chilled. Makes a delightful accompaniment to cookies. Serves four.

PUMPKIN PUDDING OR PIE FILLING

1 medium-sized pumpkin (about 5-6 pounds) or fall squash
1 tablespoon butter
$1/2$ teaspoon sea salt
2 cups apple juice
$3/4$ cup chestnut flour or 1 cup pureed chestnuts
2 tablespoons arrowroot flour starch
$1/4$ cup peanut butter (not hydrogenated)
2 teaspoon cinnamon
$1/4$ teaspoon fresh grated ginger
$1/4$ teaspoon ground cloves
$1/4$ teaspoon nutmeg

Scrub the pumpkin thoroughly. With a heavy knife, cut the pumpkin in half and scoop out the seeds, then quarter and cut into sections following the veins as a guide. Cut crosswise into 1-inch cubes. Heat butter in a large, heavy skillet or pot and sauté the cubes over a high flame for 10 minutes. Add sea salt and juice. Bring to a boil, then cover, lower flame, and let steam for 45 minutes, or until flesh is easily pierced with a fork. If pressure cooking, cook for 15 minutes once the pressure goes up. Drain liquid and reserve; mash the pulp or put through a food mill. Return cooking liquid to pan and beat in other ingredients with a whisk. Add pureed pumpkin and cook until thick, stirring occasionally. This pudding can be either poured into a mold and chilled, or baked in an oiled casserole in a 325 degree oven for 30 minutes. For pumpkin pie, pour into a 10-minute baked pie crust and bake for another 25 minutes.

SQUASH COMPOTE

1 tablespoon butter
4 pounds butternut, buttercup, or other fall squash, cubed
2 pounds tart red apples, cored and chopped
fruit juice (apple or orange)
1 tablespoon lemon juice
1 teaspoon grated lemon rind
2/3 cup chopped almonds
1/2 teaspoon sea salt
2 teaspoon cinnamon
nutmeg (optional)

Heat butter in a large heavy skillet or pot. Sauté squash over a high flame for 5 minutes, add apples, and sauté for another 5 minutes. Add remaining ingredients to pan, cover, and steam for 30 to 40 minutes. Add a little fruit juice if the compote looks too dry. Serve warm or cold.

Foods Containing
Dried Fruits

The following recipes make use of dried fruit and may contain too much concentrated natural carbohydrates for hypoglycemics. They should only be added to the diet in very small amounts when allowable, and should always be eaten only after a high-quality meal. For people who are not obese or hypoglycemic, they are a healthful alterative to cooking with sugar or artificial sweetening.

Breads

HEALTH NUT BREAD

Bread Batter (prepare at least 8 hours in advance)
41/2 cups liquid (grain coffee or strong herbal tea)

1 cup corn meal
3 cups oat flakes
1 cup cooked grain (any cereal)
2 teaspoon sea salt
2 teaspoon spices (cinnamon, cloves, etc.)
2½ cups whole wheat flour
¼ cup bran flakes

Remaining Batter:
1 lemon
1 fertile egg
5 tart red apples
½ cup butter
1 pound coarsely chopped nuts
½ cup soybean or chestnut flour

To make bread batter, bring liquid to a boil. Pour the corn meal into a large bowl and scald with liquid. Set aside to cool. Add oat flakes to the scalded corn meal and mix well. Add grain, sea salt, and spices. Let stand for 10 minutes. Beat in the whole wheat flour and knead mixture for 10 minutes. Cover bowl with wet terry cloth and let sit undisturbed for at least 8 hours or overnight. Preheat oven to 325 degrees. Using a fine grater, grate the entire lemon. Grate the apples coarsely. Add lemon, bran flakes, beaten egg, and apples to bread batter, mixing thoroughly after each addition. Mix in remaining ingredients. Oil 2 medium-sized bread pans and fill to the top with batter. Bake for about 2½ hours, or when a wooden skewer inserted in the center comes out clean. Let cool before serving.

NATURE'S POUND CAKE

This pound cake is made with high-quality carbohydrates.

½ cup raisins or currants
2 cups apple juice

$1/4$ cup bran
1 fertile egg
$1 1/2$ cups millet flour
$1/2$ cup sweet rice or brown rice flour
$1/2$ cup chestnut flour or pureed chestnuts
$1/4$ cup sesame butter or nut butter
$1/2$ teaspoon sea salt
$1/2$ teaspoon coriander
dash nutmeg
$1/2$ cup chopped almonds or walnuts

Preheat oven to 350 degrees. Simmer raisins in apple juice in a covered saucepan. Puree raisins, bran, egg, and liquid in a blender. Beat in remaining ingredients except for nuts. Fold in nuts and pour into an oiled 9x5x3$1/2$-inch bread pan and bake for 1 hour.

FIRESIDE COOKIES

3 cups oat flakes
2 cups boiling fruit juice
2 fertile eggs
$1/2$ cup chestnut flour or $1/4$ cup each soybean flour and
    rice flour
$1/2$ cup whole wheat pastry flour
$1/4$ cup chopped walnuts or sunflower seeds
2 tablespoons sesame seeds
2 tablespoons butter, melted
$1/2$ teaspoon sea salt
$1 1/2$ teaspoons cinnamon
1 teaspoon vanilla or almond extract
$1/2$ cup chopped dates, figs, or raisins
1 tablespoon bran flakes

Preheat oven to 375 degrees. Pour flakes into a mixing bowl and scald with hot liquid. Let flakes sit for about 5 to 10 minutes to absorb liquid. Beat in remaining ingredients.

Brush a cookie sheet with butter, drop batter using a table-spoon, and flatten with a wet fork. Bake for 15 to 20 minutes.

GEORGIA PEANUT BUTTER BARS

batter for Fireside Cookies (above)
1 cup natural peanut butter (not hydrogenated and with no additives)
1 fertile egg
1/2 teaspoon coriander

Preheat oven to 375 degrees. Mix all ingredients together and spread out on a buttered cookie sheet with a spatula. Bake for 25 to 30 minutes and cut into bars while still warm. *Variations:* Use 1 cup Valencia peanuts and omit chopped nuts and sesame seeds. For carob peanut butter bars, replace 1/4 cup of the whole wheat pastry flour with carob flour.

DESERT PUDDING

3 cups apple (or any other fruit) juice
1 cup raw couscous
1/2 cup chopped walnuts or almonds
1/2 teaspoon sea salt
4 tablespoons peanut butter

Bring fruit juice to a boil in a 2-quart saucepan. Add remaining ingredients, bring to a boil again, and simmer for 2 minutes, stirring constantly. Cover and turn off heat. Let sit undisturbed for 15 minutes. May be served warm or cold.

LEBANESE BLUEBERRY SURPRISE

1 pint fresh blueberries
1 cup fruit juice
1 tablespoon lemon juice

2 tablespoons arrowroot flour starch
1 tablespoon bran flakes
4 cups cooked Desert Pudding (above)
$\frac{1}{2}$ teaspoon allspice

Preheat oven to 375 degrees. Rinse blueberries in cold water. Bring blueberries, fruit juice, and lemon juice to a boil in a saucepan. Remove some of the liquid and use to dissolve the starch. Add starch and bran flakes to blueberries, stirring constantly. Remove from heat when thick. Spread the bottom of a cake pan with a layer of pudding. Pour over blueberries, then remaining pudding, and cover with blueberries. Sprinkle with allspice. Bake in oven for 25 minutes.

STEAMED AUTUMN PUDDING

3 tablespoons soybean flour
1 cup apple juice
$1\frac{1}{2}$ cups water
$\frac{1}{2}$ teaspoon sea salt
3 tablespoons sesame butter
2 tablespoons bran flakes
1 teaspoon vanilla extract
$2\frac{1}{2}$ cups cooked grain, any cereal (brown rice, kasha, millet, etc.)
$1\frac{1}{2}$ cups chopped walnuts
1 tablespoon grated tangerine or orange rind
$\frac{1}{2}$ teaspoon nutmeg
2 teaspoons cinnamon

Preheat oven to 350 degrees. In a saucepan, combine soybean flour, apple juice, water, and sea salt. Bring to a boil, cover pan, and simmer for 15 minutes. Beat in sesame butter. Mix in other ingredients. Use a wooden spoon to separate grains if cereal is somewhat solidified. Transfer pudding mixture to an oiled casserole, cover, and bake for 45 minutes. Remove cover and bake for another 10 minutes. Serve warm.

SETTLER'S PUDDING

3 cups oat bran or rice bran
4 cups grain coffee or apple juice
$1/2$ teaspoon sea salt
2 tablespoons soybean flour or chestnut flour
2 tablespoons arrowroot flour starch
1 cup cooked grain (any cereal)
$1/2$ cup crushed nuts
2 teaspoons cinnamon
$1/4$ teaspoon nutmeg
Soy Cream Sauce (optional; see page 238)

Preheat oven to 350 degrees. Put bran into a mixing bowl. In a saucepan bring liquid and sea salt to a boil and simmer for 10 minutes. Pour hot liquid over the bran and mix well. Beat in flours, cooked grain, nuts, and spices. Pour pudding into a buttered 2-quart casserole and cover. Bake for 2 hours; remove cover during the last 30 minutes of baking. May be served with cream or a sauce.

GAELIC SPIRAL BREAD

The spiral design of this bread appears when you cut the bread into serving pieces.

1 cup brown rice flour
1 cup yellow corn flour
4 cups apple juice
1 small sliced apple
$1/2$ teaspoon sea salt
$11/2$ cups whole wheat pastry flour
$1/4$ cup bran flakes
$1/4$ cup soybean flour

1 fertile egg, beaten
1/2 cup chopped nuts
1 1/2 tablespoons cinnamon
4 tablespoons any natural nut butter
2 tablespoons fruit juice
grated lemon or orange rind (optional)

Put rice and corn flours into a large mixing bowl and set aside. Bring the 4 cups liquid to a boil with the apple. Cover and simmer for 5 minutes. Holding a strainer over the mixing bowl, pour the hot liquid over the flours. Mix flours thoroughly with a wooden spoon until all the liquid is absorbed. Then add the sea salt, pastry flour, bran flakes, and soybean flour and mix again. In a separate bowl, mix together the beaten egg, nuts, cinnamon, nut butter, juice, and rind. Spread the dough out on a well-floured (use soy flour) breadboard and flatten to about 1-inch thickness. Coat the entire surface of the dough with the mixture filling and roll up, like a jelly roll. Transfer bread to a well-buttered pan and make a few slashes across the top with a sharp knife. Cover bread with a damp cloth and place in a warm spot for a couple of hours. Preheat oven to 350 degrees. Bake for 40 minutes with a covering of tin foil. Remove foil and bake for another 30 to 40 minutes, or until lightly browned.

FIBER MUFFINS

2 cups wheat or rice bran
1 cup whole wheat pastry flour
2 tablespoons soybean flour
2 teaspoons cinnamon
1/2 teaspoon sea salt
2 tablespoons sesame seeds
2 tablespoons melted butter
1 cup apple juice
1/2 cup currants or chopped dried fruit

2 cups cooked cereal (any grain)
1 fertile egg, beaten

Preheat oven to 350 degrees and insert empty muffin tins. Mix bran with flours, cinnamon, sea salt, sesame seeds, and butter until mixture is fine and crumbly. Bring apple juice to a boil in a saucepan and add fruit. Simmer for a few minutes. Pour liquid immediately over the bran mixture. Mix batter lightly and let stand for a few minutes. Then mix in cooked cereal and beaten eggs and knead thoroughly for 5 minutes. Remove muffin tins from oven and brush wells with oil. Fill muffin tins to the top and bake for 50 to 60 minutes.

ALADDIN'S CRUNCHIES

2/3 cup currants or chopped dried fruit
2 cups fruit juice
2/3 cup corn flour
1/3 cup soybean flour
1 cup whole wheat pastry flour
1/2 cup brown rice flour or barley flour
2 fertile eggs
1/4 cup butter
2 teaspoon cinnamon
1/2 teaspoon sea salt
1 cup sesame seeds
2 tablespoons bran flakes

Preheat oven to 375 degrees. Bring currants and fruit juice to a boil in a saucepan and simmer for 5 minutes. Pour corn flour into a mixing bowl and, holding a strainer over the bowl, scald corn flour with cooking liquid. Mix thoroughly. Puree the cooked fruit in a blender or food mill. Add to corn flour and mix in remaining ingredients. Butter a shallow cake pan or cookie sheet and spread out batter with a spatula to about ½-inch thickness. Bake for 15 to 20 minutes. Cut into squares while cookies are still warm.

FRUIT TREAT

⅓ cup whole wheat pastry flour
2½ cups oat flakes
1 tablespoon soybean flour
2 teaspoons cinnamon
½ teaspoon sea salt
½ cup butter
1 orange
6 large apples (or pears, peaches, etc.), cored, and sliced
  into eighths
½ cup chopped dried fruit
½ cup chopped walnuts or almonds
2 teaspoons nutmeg

Preheat oven to 375 degrees. Mix dry ingredients together in a bowl. Add melted butter and rub into mixture with your fingers until crumbly. Cut the orange in half and squeeze juice over the oat mixture. Press about ⅓ of the oat mixture into a shallow cake pan. Arrange a layer of the apples and some of the dried fruit and nuts. Repeat until all the apples and oat crumbs are used up. Cover pan tightly with foil. Bake for 40 minutes. Remove cover and place under the broiler for a few minutes until the top is brown.

MOCK MINCEMEAT PIE

½ cup soybeans
1 cup dried apples
½ cup dried pears
4-5 cups water
2 teaspoons cinnamon
¼ teaspoon nutmeg
½ teaspoon ground ginger

$1/2$ teaspoon sea salt
$1/2$ cup chopped walnuts
2 tablespoons nut butter
rye or whole wheat piecrust

Place beans, dried fruit, water, and cinnamon in a large, heavy saucepan or pressure cooker. If pressure cooking, use only 4 cups of water. Pressure cook for 45 minutes once pressure goes up. For regular cooking, use 5 cups of water, bring ingredients to a boil, and then cover, lower flame, and simmer for 2 hours. Preheat oven to 350 degrees. Prepare piecrust and place in a 9-inch diameter pan. Bake for 10 minutes and remove from oven. Puree soybean filling and mix in remaining ingredients. Spoon into piecrust and cover with thin strips of leftover pie dough. Bake for 40 minutes.

PILGRIM BREAD PUDDING

3 cups cubed whole-grain bread
2 cups grain coffee
$1/2$ cup currants or chopped dried fruit
2 teaspoons ground cinnamon
$1/2$ teaspoon sea salt
1 tablespoon grated lemon or orange rind
2 fertile eggs, beaten
3 pears or apples, chopped
$1/2$ cup chopped nuts
$1/2$ cup wheat germ or bran
2 cups Vanilla Sauce or Soy Cream Sauce (see following recipes)

Soak bread crumbs in grain coffee with currants, cinnamon, sea salt, and lemon rind for several hours or overnight. Preheat oven to 350 degrees. Add beaten eggs, apples, and nuts to pudding mixture. Butter a casserole dish and sprinkle with some of the wheat germ. Spoon pudding into the casserole dish and top with remaining wheat germ. Cover dish and bake for 45 minutes. Remove cover and bake for another 10 minutes. Serve hot with chilled vanilla sauce or soy cream sauce.

VANILLA SAUCE

This sauce may be served alone as a pudding, but it goes well over any dessert.

$\frac{1}{2}$ cup sesame butter (tahini)
$\frac{1}{2}$ cup sweet rice flour
$\frac{1}{8}$ teaspoon sea salt
1 teaspoon pure vanilla extract
3 cups apple juice

Pour oil off the top of the sesame butter and pour into a saucepan. If there is no excess oil, use 2 tablespoons sesame oil. Heat oil over a low flame and add flour. Sauté for a few minutes and remove from heat. Add remaining ingredients and beat with a whisk to eliminate lumps. Bring sauce to a boil over a medium heat, lower flame and simmer uncovered for 30 minutes, stirring occasionally. Sauce is ready to use warm, or it may be chilled and whipped for a lighter consistency.

SOY CREAM SAUCE

This cream sauce is good over any dessert.

2 tablespoons soybean flour
$2\frac{1}{4}$ cups apple juice
1 lemon
1 heaping tablespoon arrowroot flour starch
1 teaspoon pure vanilla extract
2 tablespoons butter
dash of sea salt

Dissolve soybean flour in 2 cups apple juice in a saucepan. Bring to a boil, and stir constantly until thick. This should be done over an asbestos pad or double boiler because soybean flour burns easily. After about 5 minutes, cut the lemon in half and squeeze about 1 tablespoon of juice into arrowroot. Add remaining apple juice and mix into a paste. Stir arrowroot mixture into sauce and cook for another 5 minutes, stirring constantly. Remove from the stove and let cool for a few minutes. Grate a teaspoon of lemon rind into the sauce. Add vanilla. Heat butter in a separate pan. Pour sauce into a blender or deep bowl and beat until foamy. Add sea salt and slowly add the butter, a drop at a time, and continue beating until sauce is smooth. Serve over warm dessert, or chill in the freezer and serve as a custard over cooked fruit, cookies, etc.

POW-WOW PUDDING

3 cups apple juice
1/2 cup chopped dried fruits
2/3 cup white corn meal
2 apples, grated
1/2 cup chopped nuts
4 tablespoons soybean flour
2 tablespoons butter
1/2 teaspoon sea salt
2 teaspoons cinnamon
2 fertile eggs, beaten

Preheat oven to 350 degrees. Bring apple juice to a boil and add dried fruit. Cover and simmer for 15 minutes. Pour corn meal into a mixing bowl and scald with hot apple juice. Stir quickly to prevent lumping. Let cool for a few minutes before beating in other ingredients. Bake for 1 hour in a buttered casserole. Serve either hot or cold.

ST. JOHN'S BROWNIES

1/2 cup carob powder, plain (no sugar added)
2 cups apple juice

2 teaspoons vanilla extract
1 cup whole wheat pastry flour
$1/2$ cup buckwheat flour or rye flour
2 tablespoons soybean flour
1 cup pureed chestnuts (optional)
$1/4$ teaspoon cinnamon
$1/2$ teaspoon sea salt
$1/2$ teaspoon coriander
$1/2$ cup chopped nuts
$1/2$ cup currants or chopped dates
$1/4$ cup butter
2 fertile eggs
2 tablespoons bran flakes

Preheat oven to 350 degrees. Place carob powder in a saucepan. Beat in apple juice with a wire whisk. Combine all ingredients together in a mixing bowl. Pour batter into a well-buttered 9x15x2$1/2$-inch cake pan. Bake for 1 hour and 15 minutes, or until the top is dark and firm to the touch. Cut into 28 2-inch squares.

Reading Recommendations

BODY, MIND, AND SUGAR
by E. M. Abrahamson and A. W. Pezet
Holt, Rinehart & Winston, New York, 1951
(also in paperback from Pyramid Books)

BODY, MIND, AND THE B VITAMINS
by Ruth Adams and Frank Murray
Larchmont Books, New York, 1972

THE CANCER ANSWER II
by Maureen Salaman
Statford Publishers, Menlo Park, California, 1995

CANDIDA
by Luc De Schepper, M.D.
De Schepper Publishing, Santa Monica, California, 1990

CONSUMER BEWARE
by Beatrice Trum Hunter
Bantam Books, New York, 1971

COOKING CREATIVELY WITH NATURAL FOODS
by Edith and Sam Brown
Hawthorn Publishers, New York, 1972

THE DIET BIBLE
by Maureen Salaman
Statford Publishers, Menlo Park, California, 1994

DIET FOR A SMALL PLANET
by Frances Moore Lappé
Ballantine Books, Inc., New York, 1971

DR. MARCUS LAUX'S NATURALLY WELL, HEALING
WITH THE POWER OF NATURE
(newsletter)
7811 Montrose Road
Potomac, Maryland, 20854

DR. ROBERT ATKINS' HEALTH REVEALATIONS
(newsletter)
105 Monument Street
Baltimore, Maryland, 21201

EATING RIGHT FOR YOU
by Carlton Fredericks
Grosset and Dunlap, New York, 1972

ENTER THE ZONE
by Barry Sears, Ph.D.
HarperCollins, New York, 1995

FEED YOUR KIDS RIGHT
by Lendon Smith, M.D.
McGraw-Hill, New York, 1979

FIGHTING DEPRESSION
by Harvey Ross, M.D.
Larchmont Books, New York, 1975

FOODS THAT HEAL
by Maureen Salaman
Statford Publishers, Menlo Park, California, 1989

GOODBYE ALLERGIES
by Judge Tom R. Blaine
Citadel Press, Secaucus, New Jersey, 1965

HEALTH AND LIGHT
by John Ott, Sc.D.
Devin-Adair Co., Old Greenwich, Conn., 1973

HEALTH FREEDOM NEWS
(magazine)
The National Health Federation
P.O. Box 688
Monrovia, California, 91017
Tel: (818) 357-2181   Fax: (818) 303-0642

HUNZA HEALTH SECRETS
by Renee Taylor
Prentice Hall, Englewood Cliffs, N.J., 1964

HYPOGLYCEMIA: A BETTER APPROACH
by Paavo Airola, Ph.D.
Health Plus, Publishers,
Phoenix, Arizona, 1977

HYPOGLYCEMIA
YOUR BONDAGE OR FREEDOM
by Richard Barmakian
Altura Health Publishers, Irvine, California, 1976

JOURNAL OF OPTIMAL NUTRITION
2546 Regis Drive
Davis, California, 95616

LOW BLOOD SUGAR AND YOU
by Carlton Fredericks and Herman Goodman
Grosset and Dunlap, New York, 1969

THE LOW BLOOD SUGAR COOKBOOK
by Margo Blevinand and Geri Ginder
Doubleday and Co., Inc., Garden City, N.Y., 1973

LOW BLOOD SUGAR GOURMET COOKBOOK
by Sylvia C. L. Dannett with Maureen McCabe
Drake Publisher, Inc., New York, 1974

MEGA-NUTRIENTS
by Dr. Herbert Newhold
Wyden Publications, New York, 1975

THE NATURAL FOODS SWEET-TOOTH COOKBOOK
by Eunice Farmitant
Doubleday and Co., Inc., Garden City, N.Y., 1973

A NEW BREED OF DOCTOR
by Alan H. Nittler, M.D.
Pyramid Books, New York, 1972

NUTRITION AND ALCOHOLISM
by Roger Williams, M.D.
University of Oklahoma Press,
Norman, Oklahoma, 1951

NUTRITION FOR TOTS TO TEENS
(and all other ages)
by Emory W. Thurston, Ph.D., SCD
Argold Press, Inc.,
Encino, California

NUTRITION, THE CANCER ANSWER
By Maureen Salaman
Statford Publishers, Menlo Park, California, 1984

PLEASE, DOCTOR, DO SOMETHING
by Joe D. Nichols, M.D.
Natural Food Associates,
Atlanta, Texas, 1972

PREVENTION
(magazine published monthly)
by Rodale Press, Inc.
Emmaus, Pa.

THE PSYCHO-METABOLIC BLUES
by Jerome Marmourstein, M.D., and Nanette Marmourstein
Woodbridge Press, Santa Barbara, Ca., 1979

RECIPES FOR A SMALL PLANET
by Ellen Buchman Ewald
Ballantine Books, Inc., New York, 1973

SUGAR BLUES
by William Dufty
Warner Books, New York, 1975

SUPER NUTRITION
by Richard Passwater
Dial Press, New York, 1975

THE SUPERMARKET HANDBOOK
by Nikki and David Goldbeck
Plume Books, New York, 1973

VITAMIN E FOR AILING AND HEALTHY HEARTS
by Dr. Wilfrid E. Shute
Pyramid Books, New York, 1969

THE YEAST CONNECTION
by William G. Crook, M.D.
Professional Books, Jackson, Tennessee, 1991

THE YEAST CONNECTION AND THE WOMAN
by William G. Crook, M.D.
Professional Books, Jackson, Tennessee, 1991

THE YEAST CONNECTION COOKBOOK
by William G. Crook, M.D. and Marjorie Hurt Jones, R.N.
Professional Books, Jackson, Tennessee, 1991

THE YEAST SYNDROME
by John Trowbridge, M.D. and Morton Walker, D.P.M.
Bantam Books, New York, 1986

About the Authors

Jeraldine Saunders is a well known nutrition writer, world-wide lecturer, consultant and an active member of the Institute for the Study of Optimal Nutrition.

Harvey M. Ross, M.D., a prominent Board Certified Psychiatrist, is a Founding Fellow and President Emeritus of the Academy of Orthomolecular Psychiatry and Past President of the International College of Applied Nutrition, and Trustee of The Huxley Institute of Biosocial Research. Dr. Ross is now retired.